T0261622

Emergency Triage

Manchester Triage Group

Emergency Triage

Manchester Triage Group

EDITED BY

Kevin Mackway-Jones

Janet Marsden

Jill Windle

THIRD EDITION
(Version 3.8)

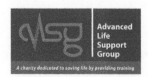

WILEY Blackwell

This edition first published 2014 © 2014 by John Wiley & Sons, Ltd. This version updated 2023 (Version 3.8)
Second edition 2006 © Blackwell Publishing Ltd.
First edition 1997 © BMJ Publishing Group

Registered office: John Wiley & Sons, Ltd, The Atrium, Southern Gate, Chichester,
West Sussex, PO19 8SQ, UK

Editorial offices: 9600 Garsington Road, Oxford, OX4 2DQ, UK
111 River Street, Hoboken, NJ 07030-5774, USA

For details of our global editorial offices, for customer services and for information about how to apply for
permission to reuse the copyright material in this book please see our website at
www.wiley.com/wiley-blackwell

The right of the author to be identified as the author of this work has been asserted in accordance with the
UK Copyright, Designs and Patents Act 1988.

All rights reserved. No part of this publication may be reproduced, stored in a retrieval system, or
transmitted, in any form or by any means, electronic, mechanical, photocopying, recording or otherwise,
except as permitted by the UK Copyright, Designs and Patents Act 1988, without the prior permission of the
publisher.

Designations used by companies to distinguish their products are often claimed as trademarks. All brand
names and product names used in this book are trade names, service marks, trademarks or registered
trademarks of their respective owners. The publisher is not associated with any product or vendor
mentioned in this book. It is sold on the understanding that the publisher is not engaged in rendering
professional services. If professional advice or other expert assistance is required, the services of a competent
professional should be sought.

The contents of this work are intended to further general scientific research, understanding, and discussion
only and are not intended and should not be relied upon as recommending or promoting a specific method,
diagnosis, or treatment by health science practitioners for any particular patient. The publisher and the
author make no representations or warranties with respect to the accuracy or completeness of the contents
of this work and specifically disclaim all warranties, including without limitation any implied warranties of
fitness for a particular purpose. In view of ongoing research, equipment modifications, changes in
governmental regulations, and the constant flow of information relating to the use of medicines,
equipment, and devices, the reader is urged to review and evaluate the information provided in the package
insert or instructions for each medicine, equipment, or device for, among other things, any changes in the
instructions or indication of usage and for added warnings and precautions. Readers should consult with a
specialist where appropriate. The fact that an organization or Website is referred to in this work as a citation
and/or a potential source of further information does not mean that the author or the publisher endorses
the information the organization or Website may provide or recommendations it may make. Further,
readers should be aware that Internet Websites listed in this work may have changed or disappeared
between when this work was written and when it is read. No warranty may be created or extended by any
promotional statements for this work. Neither the publisher nor the author shall be liable for any damages
arising herefrom.

Library of Congress Cataloging-in-Publication Data

Emergency triage / Manchester Triage Group; edited by Kevin Mackway-Jones, Janet Marsden, Jill Windle.
Third edition.
    p. ; cm.
    Includes bibliographical references and index.
    ISBN 978-1-118-29906-7 (pbk.: alk. paper) – ISBN 978-1-118-29902-9 – ISBN 978-1-118-29903-6
(emobi) – ISBN 978-1-118-29904-3 (epdf) – ISBN 978-1-118-29905-0 (epub)
    I. Mackway-Jones, Kevin, editor. II. Marsden, Janet, editor. III. Windle, Jill, editor. IV. Manchester
Triage Group, issuing body.
    [DNLM: 1. Triage methods. 2. Emergency Service, Hospital. WX 215]
    RA975.5.E5
    362.18–dc23
                                                                                              2013024786

A catalogue record for this book is available from the British Library.

Wiley also publishes its books in a variety of electronic formats. Some content that appears in print may not
be available in electronic books.

Anyone wishing to license all or part of this book in electronic format for integration into a software
product or a hospital's electronic patient records, or anyone wishing to license this title for translation please
contact alsg@wiley.com

Cover design by Nathan Harris

Set in 9.5/13pt Meridien by Aptara® Inc., New Delhi, India
Printed and bound by CPI Group (UK) Ltd, Croydon, CR0 4YY

C9781118299067_310724

Contents

Editors

Kevin Mackway-Jones, Consultant Emergency Physician, Manchester Royal Infirmary and Royal Manchester Children's Hospital; Medical Director, North West Ambulance Service; Honorary Civilian Consultant Advisor in Emergency Medicine to the British Army; Professor of Emergency Medicine, Centre for Effective Emergency Care, Manchester Metropolitan University.

Janet Marsden, Professor of Ophthalmology and Emergency Care and Director, Centre for Effective Emergency Care, Manchester Metropolitan University.

Jill Windle, Lecturer Practitioner in Emergency Nursing, Salford Royal Hospitals NHS Foundation Trust and University of Salford.

Members of the original Manchester Triage Group

Kassim Ali, Consultant in Emergency Medicine

Simon Brown, Senior Emergency Nurse

Helen Fiveash, Senior Emergency Nurse

Julie Flaherty, Senior Paediatric Emergency Nurse

Stephanie Gibson, Senior Emergency Nurse

Chris Lloyd, Senior Emergency Nurse

Kevin Mackway-Jones, Consultant in Emergency Medicine

Sue McLaughlin, Senior Paediatric Emergency Nurse

Janet Marsden, Senior Ophthalmic Emergency Nurse

Rosemary Morton, Consultant in Emergency Medicine

Karen Orry, Senior Emergency Nurse

Barbara Phillips, Consultant in Paediatric Emergency Medicine

Phil Randall, Consultant in Emergency Medicine

Joanne Royle, Senior Emergency Nurse

Brendan Ryan, Consultant in Emergency Medicine

Ian Sammy, Consultant in Emergency Medicine

Steve Southworth, Consultant in Emergency Medicine

Debbie Stevenson, Senior Emergency Nurse

Claire Summers, Consultant in Emergency Medicine

Jill Windle, Lecturer Practitioner in Emergency Nursing

International Reference Group

Austria
Stefan Kovacevic
Andreas Lueger
Willibald Pateter

Brazil
Welfane Cordeiro
Maria do Carmos Rausch
Bárbara Torres

Germany
Joerg Krey
Heinzpeter Moecke
Peter Niebuhr

Mexico
Alfredo Tanaka Chavez
Elizabeth Hernandez Delgadillo
Noe Arellano Hernandez

Norway
Grethe Doelbakken
Endre Sandvik
Germar Schneider

Portugal
Paulo Freitas
Antonio Marques
Angela Valenca

Spain
Gabriel Redondo Torres
Juan Carlos Medina Álvarez
Gema García Riestra

Preface to the third edition

Time continues to move on and it is now nearly 20 years since a group of senior emergency physicians and emergency nurses first met to consider solutions to the muddle that was triage in Manchester, UK. We had no expectation that the solution to our local problems would be robust enough (and timely enough) to become the triage solution for the whole United Kingdom. Never in our wildest dreams did we imagine that the Manchester Triage System (MTS) would be generic enough to be adopted around the world. Much to our surprise, however, both of these fantastic ideas came about, and the MTS continues to be used in many languages to triage tens of millions of Emergency Department attenders each year.

The basic principles that drive the MTS (recognition of the presentation and reductive discriminator identification) are unchanging – but from time to time it has become necessary to make some adjustments to the detail. The third edition builds on the changes we made in the second; it takes into account the comments passed to us by users over the years (for which we are very grateful) and also the contributions of the International Reference Group, who bring a broad perspective from other clinical situations and cultures. It also seeks to include modifications that reflect new research and alterations in the practice of emergency care. Significant changes include new charts for unwell neonates and babies and a major, evidence-based change in the way in which fever in childhood is prioritised. We have clarified discriminator terminology and definitions where this was proving difficult (for instance 'abnormal pulse' is now clarified as 'new abnormal pulse' and 'known immunosupression' has been restated as 'known or likely immunospression'). We have also taken the opportunity to standardise the order in which discriminators appear on the charts. Overall though, as in the second edition, the changes are small in number.

This new edition also continues our attempt to put triage in the context of changes that are happening in many emergency care systems around the world. Emergency care continues to be the focus of political and management attention. The care of increasing numbers of patients with less urgent conditions (who make up the majority in most settings) continue to be a source of concern, since under-resourced systems that focused (rightly) on patients with the highest clinical priority inevitably resulted in delayed care for those at the other end of the priority scale. In the consumer age, this delay (which delivers a poor patient experience) is unacceptable. It is often easier to blame the clinical prioritisation system (triage) for this delay than to deal with an under-resourced system. Another current vogue is to try to replace a dedicated emergency care triage system with a hospital-wide track and trigger score. The evidence is clear that, unsurprisingly, this cannot be done without a considerable additional risk to physiologically normal patients early in the evolution of their illness.

Our standpoint has always been that proper emergency triage is vital in all systems or circumstances where the demand for emergency care outstrips the ability to deliver it. We continue to believe that these circumstances occur occasionally in even the best managed and resourced systems, and frequently in those with the usual demands and staffing. Thus clinical prioritisation (whether called triage, initial assessment or anything else) remains a cornerstone of clinical risk management in emergency care, and abandoning it completely is not an option.

Kevin Mackway-Jones, Janet Marsden, Jill Windle
Manchester, 2013

Preface to the first edition

Every day, emergency departments are faced with a large number of patients suffering from a wide range of problems. The workload varies from day to day and from hour to hour and depends on the number of patients attending and what is wrong with them. It is absolutely essential that there is a system in place to ensure that these patients are seen in order of clinical need, rather than in order of attendance.

In the past year great steps have been made towards establishing a National Triage Scale in the United Kingdom; this follows on from similar work in Australia and Canada. This book is intended to allow practitioners of triage to work to a set standard when applying national scales to the patients presenting to their departments. The members of the multi-professional consensus group that designed this methodology hope that individual practitioners will use it to inform the triage process and ensure that their decisions are both valid and reproducible.

This manual contains the basic knowledge necessary for triage practitioners to begin to build their competence in performing triage. It is hoped that practitioners will find a useful source reference and *aide-memoire*.

Kevin Mackway-Jones, 1996

CHAPTER 1
Introduction

Background

Triage is a system of clinical risk management employed in Emergency Departments worldwide to manage patient flow safely when clinical need exceeds capacity. Systems are intended to ensure care is defined according to patient need and in a timely manner. Early Emergency Department triage was intuitive, rather than methodological, and was therefore neither reproducible between practitioners nor auditable.

The Manchester Triage Group was first set up in November 1994 with the aim of establishing consensus among senior emergency nurses and emergency physicians about triage standards. It soon became apparent that the Group's aims could be set out under five headings.

- Development of the common nomenclature
- Development of common definitions
- Development of a robust triage methodology
- Development of a training package
- Development of an audit guide for triage

Nomenclature and definitions

A review of the triage nomenclature and definitions that were in use at the time revealed considerable differences. A representative sample of these is summarised in Table 1.1, where the priority categories are shown on the left and the maximum respective times (in minutes) to first contact by a treating clinincan are listed in the right-hand columns.

Emergency Triage: Manchester Triage Group, Third Edition.
Edited by Kevin Mackway-Jones, Janet Marsden and Jill Windle.
© 2014 John Wiley & Sons, Ltd. Published 2014 by John Wiley & Sons, Ltd.

Table 1.1

Hospital 1		Hospital 2		Hospital 3			Hospital 4
Red	0	A	0	Immediate	0	1	0
Amber	<15	B	<10	Urgent	5–10	2	<10
		C	<60	Semi-urgent	30–60		
Green	<120	D	<120				
Blue	<240	E	–	Delay acceptable	–	3	–
		FGHI					

Despite this enormous variation, it was also apparent that there were a number of common themes running through the timings of these different triage systems, and these are highlighted in Table 1.2.

Table 1.2

Priority	Max. time (minutes)			
1	0	0	0	0
2	<15	<10	5–10	<10
3		<60	30–60	
4	120	<120		
5	<240	–	–	–

Once the common themes of triage had been highlighted, it became possible to quickly agree on a new common nomenclature and definition system. Each of the new categories was given a number, a colour and a name and was defined in terms of ideal maximum time to first contact with the treating clinician. At meetings between representatives of Emergency Nursing and Emergency Medicine nationally, this work informed the derivation of the United Kingdom triage scale shown in Table 1.3.

Table 1.3

Number	Name	Colour	Max. time (minutes)
1	Immediate	Red	0
2	Very urgent	Orange	10
3	Urgent	Yellow	60
4	Standard	Green	120
5	Non-urgent	Blue	240

As practice has developed over the past 20 years, five-part triage scales have been established around the world. The target times themselves are locally set, being influenced by politics as much as by medicine, particularly at lower priorities, but the concept of varying clinical priority remains current.

Triage methodology

In general terms a triage method can try and provide the practitioner with the diagnosis, with the disposal or with a clinical priority. The Triage Group quickly decided that the triage methodology should be designed to allocate a clinical priority. This decision was based on three major tenets. First, the aim of the triage encounter in an Emergency Department is to aid both clinical management of the individual patient and departmental management; this is best achieved by accurate allocation of a clinical priority. Second, the length of the triage encounter is such that any attempts to accurately diagnose a patient are doomed to fail, as this activity requires a consultation rather than a triage assessment. Finally, it is apparent that diagnosis is not accurately linked to clinical priority, the latter reflects a number of aspects of the particular patient's presentation as well as the diagnosis; for example, patients with a final diagnosis of ankle sprain may present with severe, moderate or no pain, and their clinical priority must reflect this.

In outline, the triage method put forward in this book requires practitioners to select from a range of presentations, and then to seek a limited number of signs and symptoms at each level of clinical priority. The signs and symptoms that discriminate between the clinical priorities are termed *discriminators* and they are set out in the form of flow charts for each presentation – the *presentational flow charts*. Discriminators that indicate higher levels of priority are sought first, and to a large degree patients who are allocated to the standard / 4 / green clinical priority are selected by default.

The decision-making process is discussed in chapter 2, and the triage method itself is explained in detail in chapter 3.

Priority and management

It is easy to become confused between the clinical priority and the clinical management of a patient. The former requires that enough information is gathered to enable the patient to be placed into one of the five defined categories as discussed above. The latter may well require a much deeper understanding of the patient's needs, and may be affected by a large number of extraneous factors, such as the time of day, the state of the staffing and the number of beds available. Furthermore, the availability of services for particular patients will fundamentally affect individual patient flow. Separately staffed 'streams' of care for particular patient groups will run at different rates. This does not affect underlying clinical priority which affects the order of care within, rather than between, streams in such a system. These issues are discussed in more detail in chapter 5.

Training for triage

This book, in conjunction with the accompanying Manchester Triage Provider Course, attempts to provide the training necessary to allow introduction of a standard triage method. This process has been highly successful, not only in the UK where the system originated, but across many countries that sought a standard for triage in their health care systems. It is not envisaged that reading the book and attending a course can produce instant expertise in triage. Rather, this process will introduce the method and allow practitioners to develop competence at using the material available as a first step towards competence in using the system. It must be followed up by audit of individual triage practitioners and evaluation of their use of the system.

Triage audit

The Triage Group spent considerable time trying to pin down 'sentinel diagnoses' – that is diagnoses that could be identified retrospectively and which could be used as markers of accurate triage. For the reasons outlined above, it soon became apparent that even retrospective diagnosis could not accurately predict actual clinical priority at presentation.

Successful introduction of a robust audit method is essential to the future of any standard methodology, since reproducibility between individual practitioners and departments must be shown to exist. This is discussed in more detail in chapter 6.

Beyond triage in the Emergency Department

The concept of triage (determining clinical need as a method of managing clinical risk) and the process outlined in this book (presentational recognition followed by reductive discriminator seeking) is applicable in other settings. In some of these, for example medical, surgical or paediatric assessment units, the system can be implemented in exactly the same way as it is in the Emergency Department. In other settings, for instance Primary Care or Out of Hours Units, many contacts may be made by telephone. A modification of the Manchester Triage System (MTS) can be used and this is outlined in chapter 7.

The information gained during the triage process can also be used in other ways to improve patient care. It is important, for instance, that clinicians recognise any change in the patients' status as early as possible. Early Warning Scores have been applied in many settings to formalise this function. In the Emergency Department the ABCDE discriminators from the MTS can be used in exactly this way, and the monitoring of physiological parameters, as outlined in chapter 8, is an intuitive way for triage practitioners to put into practice the original exhortation for dynamic triage and that 'every intervention is a triage intervention'.

Finally, many users of the MTS have recognised that the outcome of the presentation selection–priority assignment process is to place individual patients into one of 265 slots in a 53×5 presentation–priority matrix. This 'pigeon-holing' can be used to drive pathways of care in systems that have taken to 'streaming'. Particular presentation–priority combinations (e.g. wounds–green, chest pain–orange) may be appropriate to particular streams (minor injuries and resuscitation, respectively, in the examples given). This concept is discussed in more detail in chapter 8.

Summary

Triage is a fundamental part of clinical risk management in all departments when clinical load exceeds clinical availability. Emergency triage promulgates a system that delivers a teachable, auditable method of assigning clinical priority in emergency settings. It is not designed to judge whether patients are appropriately in the emergency setting, but to ensure that those who need care receive it appropriately quickly. MTS has been shown to have functions beyond the initial concept when used to monitor care and to signpost streams of care determined by local provision and actual availability.

CHAPTER 2

The decision-making process and triage

Introduction

Decision making is an essential and integral part of nursing and medical practice. Sound clinical judgment in relation to patient care requires both knowledge and experience. Many practitioners argue that critical decision making is only about 'common sense' and 'problem solving', and to a certain extent they are correct. It is, however, more than this and requires a high level of skill. Within the decision-making process, clinicians are expected to:

Interpret
Discriminate
Evaluate

the information they gather about patients, and critically appraise their actions following that decision. Without a framework of reference on which to base these decisions, they will be unstructured, haphazard and potentially unsafe. The ability to make sound decisions is essential for safe and effective patient management.

Early triage systems structured the interview but gave no guidance about the action following a decision. Thus the *outcome* of the triage process was not based on a sound methodology. Triage decisions were unique to each nurse and inherently part of their own decision-making process and such decisions are likely to be fundamentally flawed without a framework of reference. To overcome this problem, a framework of reference (methodology) for the process of triage is required and a method by which practitioners can acquire the necessary skills for its implementation.

Emergency Triage: Manchester Triage Group, Third Edition.
Edited by Kevin Mackway-Jones, Janet Marsden and Jill Windle.
© 2014 John Wiley & Sons, Ltd. Published 2014 by John Wiley & Sons, Ltd.

The development of expertise

A relationship between experience and skill acquisition has been described in which there are five stages of development:

- Novice
- Advanced beginner
- Competent
- Proficient
- Expert

As practitioners develop along this continuum, they acquire skills and learn from their experiences in practice and it is expected that their decision-making ability alters and improves. The process can be facilitated by providing a system based upon a common framework that is methodologically sound, on which decisions can be based and their effectiveness evaluated.

Decision-making strategies

A number of strategies are used in the decision-making process. These are:

- Reasoning
- Pattern recognition
- Repetitive hypothesising
- Mental representation
- Intuition

Reasoning

There are essentially two types of reasoning involved in critical thinking: inductive and deductive. Inductive reasoning is the ability to consider all possibilities, and is particularly useful for the less experienced. It involves a time-consuming process of considering all patient information collected in order to reach a sound decision about the care they require.

Deductive reasoning is the simultaneous 'weeding out' of possible solutions whilst actively collecting patient information. This strategy is often unknown or unrecognised and becomes part of expert practice. It allows the practitioner to rapidly sort relevant from irrelevant information to reach a decision.

Pattern recognition

This is the strategy most commonly used by clinicians, and is particularly important when making the rapid decisions based on limited information that are necessary during triage. Pattern recognition is a method of piecing information together in an analytical sense. Clinicians interpret the pattern of the patient's signs and symptoms by comparison with relationships and conditions from previous cases. This leads them to a decision about the patient's well-being or a potential diagnosis. The ability to use this decision-making skill develops with experience, and often appears to be intuition. Novice, proficient or competent practitioners may need to use conscious problem solving to reach a solution, while their more experienced colleagues can employ pattern recognition.

Repetitive hypothesising

Repetitive hypothesising is used by clinicians to test diagnostic reasoning. By gathering data to confirm or eliminate a hypothesis, a decision can be made. Depending on the level of expertise this method can be either inductive or deductive.

Mental representation

Mental representation is a method of simplifying the situation to provide a general picture, and allow focusing on relevant information. This strategy is often used when a problem is highly complex or overwhelming. The use of analogies helps the clinician visualise the situation by simplifying the problem and allowing a different perspective. Triage decisions need to be rapid and this method has limited use at this stage in the patient's pathway.

Intuition

Intuition is inextricably linked with expertise and is commonly seen as the ability of practitioners to solve problems with relatively few data. Intuition rarely involves conscious analysis and is often expressed as a 'gut feeling' or 'strong hunch'. Expert practitioners view situations holistically and draw on past experience. Much of their knowledge is embedded in practice and referred to as tacit, where effective decisions are made by combining knowledge with decision-making theories and intuitive thought. Many expert clinicians are unaware of the mental processes they employ in the assessment and management of patients. Although intuition has remained unmeasurable, the value to clinical practice is acknowledged and well documented.

Decision making during triage

Despite all the theories, decision making is quite simply a series of steps to reach a conclusion and consists of three main phases: (i) identification of a problem; (ii) determination of the alternatives; and (iii) selection of the most appropriate alternative. An approach to making critical decisions has been described that uses the following five steps:

---

1 Identify the problem
2 Gather and analyse information related to the solution
3 Evaluate all the alternatives and select one for implementation
4 Implement the selected alternative
5 Monitor the implementation and evaluate outcomes

This approach incorporates a number of theories and methods. When applied to triage the decisions are formed as follows.

Identify the problem

This is done by obtaining information from the patients, their carers and/or any pre-hospital care personnel. This phase allows the relevant presentational flow chart to be identified.

Gather and analyse information related to the solution

Once a flow chart has been identified this phase is facilitated since discriminators can be sought at each level. The charts facilitate rapid assessment by suggesting structured questions. Pattern recognition also plays a part at this stage.

Evaluate all the alternatives and select one for implementation

Clinicians collect significant amounts of data about the patients they deal with which is collated into their own mental database and stored in compartments for easy recall. Use of this stored information is most effective when linked to an assessment or organisational framework. The presentational flow charts provide the organisational framework to order the thought process during triage. The flow charts aid decision making by providing a structure, and, importantly, support junior staff as they develop decision-making skills.

Implement the selected alternative

There are five levels of priority (as discussed in chapter 1) and the triage practitioner tests the discriminators against the patient's presentation and allocates priority at the highest level of positive discriminator. The priority therefore depends upon the urgency of the patient's condition and, once the priority is allocated, the appropriate pathway of care begins. Triage is a dynamic process and must not be seen as an isolated incident that occurs only at the beginning of the patient's journey. The triage practitioner must use their decision-making skills and expertise to identify those patients who will require ongoing monitoring and re-triage.

Monitor the implementation and evaluate outcomes

The method of triage outlined in this book ensures that the decision is pre-determined if the correct process has been followed. The triage practitioner will therefore be able to identify how and why they reached the initial outcome (priority), conduct an accurate reassessment and subsequently confirm or change the level of priority. Accurate, reproducible decisions ensure that the whole process can be audited.

Changing current decision-making practice

For many experienced clinicians the introduction of a new framework for triage decisions poses some anxieties. It is difficult to unlearn individual methods of decision making that have developed over years of practice. However, this change should be viewed as a further refinement of their present system, providing – for the first time – a clear rationale for their decisions and an auditable system. This systematic approach will be a major contribution to the body of knowledge when used to teach junior staff, who rely so heavily on experts to inform and guide their own practice. The actual process of triage decision making presented here has been shown to be effective and adaptable to many practice settings, and has value to triage practitioners irrespective of their level of experience.

CHAPTER 3

The triage method

Introduction

The method outlined in this book is designed to allow the triage practitioner to rapidly assign a clinical priority to each patient. The system selects patients with the highest priority first without making any assumptions about the diagnosis. Emergency Departments are, to a large extent, driven by the patients' presenting signs and symptoms and this lack of focus on diagnosis is, therefore, deliberate.

Five-step process to triage decision making

1 Identify the problem
2 Gather and analyse information related to the solution
3 Evaluate all the alternatives and select one for implementation
4 Implement the selected alternative
5 Monitor the implementation and evaluate outcomes

Identifying the problem

Clinical practice is geared around the concept of a *presenting complaint* – that is the chief sign or symptom identified by the patient or carer. A list of presentations pertinent to triage is shown below.

Abdominal pain in adults	Irritable child
Abdominal pain in children	Limb problems
Abscesses and local infections	Limping child
Abuse and neglect	Major trauma
Allergy	Mental illness
Apparently drunk	Neck pain
Assault	Overdose and poisoning

(Continued)

Emergency Triage: Manchester Triage Group, Third Edition.
Edited by Kevin Mackway-Jones, Janet Marsden and Jill Windle.
© 2014 John Wiley & Sons, Ltd. Published 2014 by John Wiley & Sons, Ltd.

Asthma	Palpitations
Back pain	Pregnancy
Behaving strangely	PV (per vaginum) bleeding
Bites and stings	Rashes
Burns and scalds	Self-harm
Chemical exposure	Sexually acquired infection
Chest pain	Shortness of breath in adults
Collapse	Shortness of breath in children
Crying baby	Sore throat
Dental problems	Testicular pain
Diabetes	Torso injury
Diarrhoea and vomiting	Unwell adult
Ear problems	Unwell baby
Eye problems	Unwell child
Facial problems	Unwell newborn
Falls	Urinary problems
Fits	Worried parent
Foreign body	Wounds
Gastrointestinal (GI) bleeding	Major incidents – primary
Headache	Major incidents – secondary
Head injury	

This list of presentational flow charts covers almost all presentations to Emergency Departments. The list, charts and contents were finalised after considerable discussion and have been refined, in both this and previous editions, following changes in practice, research and international consultation. The presentations fall broadly into the categories of illness, injury, children, abnormal and unusual behaviour, and major incidents.

The first part of the triage method requires the practitioner to select the most appropriate presentational flow chart from the list. The chart identifies discriminators that allow the clinical priority to be determined.

A key feature of the method is that the charts are consistent in their approach, since it is recognised that a number of patients' chief complaints may lead to more than one presentational flow chart. For example, a patient who presents feeling generally unwell with a stiff neck and a headache will be given the same priority whether the practitioner uses the *Unwell adult, Neck pain* or *Headache* flow charts.

Gathering and analysing information

To a great extent the patient's presentation will dictate which presentational flow chart is selected. Following this selection, information must be gathered and analysed to allow the actual priority to be determined. The flow chart structures this process by showing key discriminators at each level of priority – the assessment is carried out by finding the highest level at which the answer posed by the discriminator question is positive. Discriminators are deliberately posed as questions by the triage practitioner to facilitate the process.

Discriminators

Discriminators, as their name implies, are factors that discriminate between patients, such that they allow them to be allocated to one of the five clinical priorities. They can be *general* or *specific* and are arranged in the ABCDE format. General discriminators apply to all patients irrespective of their presentation and therefore appear time and time again throughout the charts; on each occasion the general discriminators will lead the triage practitioner to allocate the same clinical priority. Specific discriminators are applicable to individual presentations or to small groups of presentations, and tend to relate to key features of particular conditions. Thus while *severe pain* is a general discriminator, *cardiac pain* and *pleuritic pain* are specific discriminators. General discriminators appear in many more charts than specific ones. All the discriminators used are defined in the discriminator dictionary at the end of the book, and the definitions of the specific ones in use on individual charts are repeated on the accompanying chart notes for ease of reference. All discriminators are reviewed for each edition. Any changes are published on the triage website at www.triagenet.net.

General discriminators are a recurring feature of the charts, and a proper understanding of them is essential to an understanding of the triage method. Six general discriminators are discussed further here:

- Life threat
- Conscious level
- Haemorrhage
- Temperature
- Pain
- Acuteness

Life threat

To a practising emergency nurse or emergency physician *life threat* is perhaps the most obvious general discriminator of all. Broadly speaking this recognises that any cessation or threat to the vital (ABC) functions places the patient in priority 1 (red).

Patients who are unable to maintain their own airway for any length of time have an insecure airway. Additionally, patients with stridor have significant airway threat – this may be an inspiratory or expiratory noise, or both. Stridor is heard best on breathing with the mouth open. Absence of breathing is defined as no respiration or respiratory effort as assessed by looking, listening and feeling for 10 seconds. Inadequacy is a more difficult concept – but in general, patients who are failing to breathe well enough to maintain adequate oxygenation have inadequate breathing. There may be an increased work of breathing, signs of inadequate breathing or exhaustion. Absence of pulses is only diagnosed after palpation over a central pulse for 5 seconds. Shock can be difficult to diagnose – the classic signs include sweating, pallor, tachycardia, hypotension and reduced conscious level.

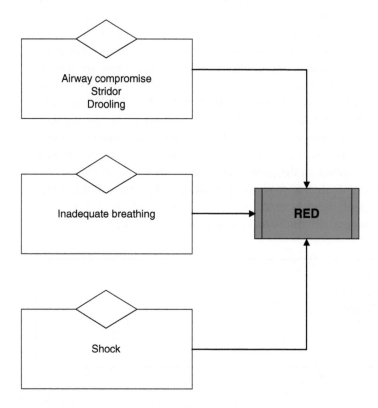

Conscious level

Conscious level is considered differently for adults and children. In adults only currently fitting patients are always categorised as priority 1 (red), while all unresponsive children are placed in this clinical priority. Adult patients with altered conscious level (responding to voice or pain or unresponsive) are categorised as priority 2 (orange), as are children who respond to voice or pain only. All patients with a history of unconsciousness should be allocated to priority 3 (yellow).

The fact that all patients with alterations in conscious level are allocated to the very urgent priority may be at odds with current practice; this is especially so with regard to the clinical priority given to patients who are intoxicated or under the influence of drugs. Two points need to be made about this. Firstly, the aetiology of alterations in level of consciousness is largely irrelevant in determining the risk to the patient – an altered conscious level due to drugs or alcohol is clinically as important as an altered conscious level due to other causes. Secondly, most drunk patients do not have an altered level of consciousness. Specific points about the allocation of clinical priority to patients who are apparently drunk are dealt with in the presentational flow chart of that name.

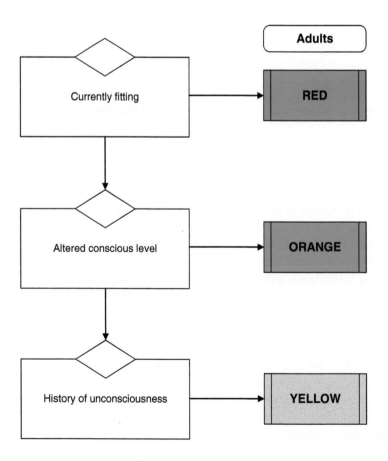

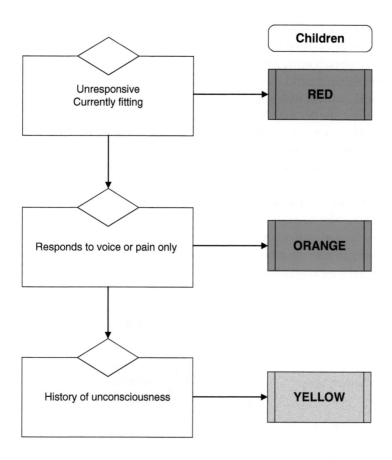

Haemorrhage

Haemorrhage is a feature of many presentations – particularly, but not exclusively, those involving trauma. The haemorrhage discriminators are exsanguinating, uncontrolled major or uncontrolled minor. The use of the success of attempts to control the haemorrhage is deliberate since, in general, continuing bleeding has a higher clinical priority. While, of course, in practice it can be difficult to decide which category a particular haemorrhage falls into, the definitions of the discriminators are designed to help the practitioner to do this. Exsanguinating haemorrhage is present if death will ensue rapidly unless bleeding is stopped. A haemorrhage that is not rapidly controlled by the application of sustained direct pressure, and in which blood continues to flow heavily or soak through large dressings quickly, is described as an uncontrollable major haemorrhage, while that in which blood continues to flow slightly or ooze, is described as uncontrollable minor haemorrhage.

Any bleeding, however minor, will, unless another discriminator leads to the allocation of a higher clinical priority, be allocated to priority 4 (green).

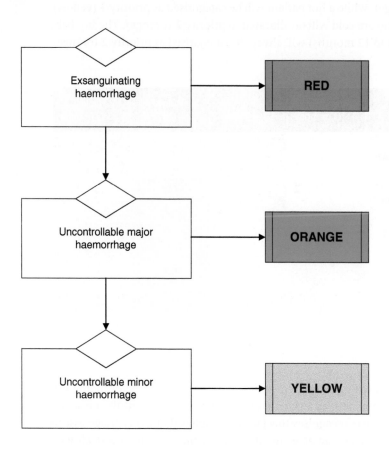

Temperature
Temperature is used as a general discriminator and accurate measurement of the temperature should be a part of the triage process, where indicated. Clinical impression of skin temperature is important and is crucial where immediate assessment of core temperature is not possible.

If the skin feels very hot, the patient is clinically said to be very hot – this corresponds to a temperature of 41°C or more; similarly if the skin feels hot the patient is clinically said to be hot and this corresponds to a temperature of 38.5°C or more. A patient with warm skin fulfils the discriminator of warmth and this goes with a temperature of less than 38.5°C.

Patients with cold skin can be said to be clinically cold – a core temperature of less than 35°C matches this.

A very hot patient (1 year and above) will always be categorised as priority 2 (orange), while a hot patient will be categorised as priority 3 (yellow). Patients who are cold will be allocated to priority 2 (orange). The hot baby (from birth to 12 months) will always be categorised as priority 2 (orange).

	Very Hot 41°C or more	Hot 38.5–40.9°C	Warm 37.5–38.4°C	Cold 35°C or less
Newborn (up to 28 days)				
Baby (child of 12 months or less)				
Child over 12 months				
Adult				

Pain

From the patient's perspective, pain is a major factor in determining priority. The use of pain as a general discriminator throughout the presentational flow charts recognises this fact and implies that every triage assessment should include an assessment of pain. Pain assessment is dealt with in chapter 4 and readers are referred there for a detailed discussion. In general terms, the discriminator severe pain is intended to imply pain that is unbearable, often described as the worst ever, while moderate pain refers to pain that is bearable but intense. Any patient with a lesser degree of recent mild pain should, if no other discriminators suggest a higher categorisation, be allocated to priority 4 (green) and not to the non-urgent category, priority 5 (blue).

The general pain discriminator describes the intensity or severity of pain only. Other characteristics of pain, such as site, radiation and periodicity, may feature as specific discriminators in particular presentational flow charts.

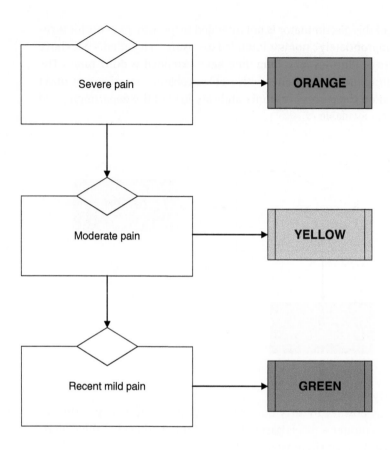

Acuteness

Within the triage method certain conventions have been used to help with consistency. The term 'abrupt' is used to indicate onset within seconds or minutes and 'acute' indicates a time period within 24 hours. Recent symptoms and signs are those that have appeared within the past 7 days.

Whilst most clinicians have no problem accepting that the acuteness of onset can help indicate the clinical priority, it is slightly more controversial to argue that chronicity (in this case greater than 7 days) is used to define a non-urgent problem. However, on reflection, it is intuitive that the relatively long time that the problem has been present indicates that the patient can be allocated the non-urgent priority without clinical risk. The triage method is such that the presence of any other general or specific discriminators relevant to the presentation will result in the allocation of a higher priority, for example, recent mild pain.

The use of this discriminator is not intended to 'punish' patients for turning up 'inappropriately', nor is it intended to ensure that patients who have had injuries or illnesses for a long time have extended waiting times. The actual waiting time for patients with stable problems not of recent onset will depend on the current case mix and case load of the department, and the resources available.

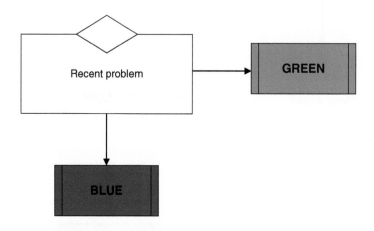

Secondary triage

It may not be possible to carry out all the assessments necessary at the initial triage encounter – this is particularly so if the workload of the department is high. In such circumstances the necessary assessments should still be carried out, but as secondary procedures by another member of the team. More time-consuming assessments (such as blood glucose estimation and peak flow measurement) are often left to the secondary stage. Many charts have a 'risk limit' placed on them, which indicates the lowest priority that can be applied to the patient if all observations needed are not complete.

Evaluating alternatives and selecting one

Selection of the most appropriate flow chart presents a number of general and specific discriminators which can then be tested against the patient. The skill in implementing the triage method lies in the application of this testing. Practitioners must decide whether the criteria for the presence of each discriminator is fulfilled, and must decide which discriminator is the most applicable at the highest clinical priority. For example, the patient who presents with neck pain following direct trauma to the neck and a pain score of 6 (both priority 3), the most appropriate discriminator is *direct trauma to the neck* as this provides more significant information about this patient.

Implementing the selected alternative

This step is essentially a procedural one. The inevitable outcome of the information gathering, analysis and evaluation leads to allocation of one of the clinical priorities shown in the Table 3.1.

Table 3.1

Number	Name	Colour
1	Immediate	Red
2	Very urgent	Orange
3	Urgent	Yellow
4	Standard	Green
5	Non-urgent	Blue

Documentation

Implementation involves recording the allocated priority and showing the decision making that led to it. The triage method outlined here allows documentation to be simple and precise. The minimum required is a record of which presentational flow chart is being used, which discriminator defines the category and which category has been selected. Thus, for instance, the triage record of a patient with chest pain might be:

Chest pain
Pleuritic pain
Urgent/priority 3 (yellow)

This simple approach to documentation allows for simple audit, but it is recognised that computer decision support software is widely used and will dictate the way the triage event is recorded.

Patient assessment

The purist view of the triage event is a rapid and focused encounter in which information is gathered and applied to assign a priority. This type of assessment is a skill in itself. The following framework can be used to teach the process to triage practitioners, ensuring decisions are based on relevant and appropriate patient data.

It is important that the assessment of a patient is systematic and all elements of that assessment are pieced together to give a complete picture of the patient's problem. For this reason the triage practitioner should have sufficient experience of emergency care and the interpersonal skills to communicate effectively with patients and their families.

The approach to this assessment should take the following format (Table 3.2):

Table 3.2

Assessment component	Triage activity
Greeting the patient	The assessment begins at first sight of the patient; watch the patient as they approach the triage area, and pick up on any visual signs, which may include: • level of mobility • obvious injury • age of patient
Patient's history	Ask the patient why they have attended the Emergency Department This is a short, concise, subjective history and tells you about the patient's injury/illness/health-related problem
Presenting complaint	The patient's presenting complaints can be established from the subjective history they provide *This leads the triage practitioner to choose the most appropriate presentation flow chart*
Focused questions (interview)	This is where the triage practitioner's knowledge and skills are most evident. Application of anatomical knowledge, pattern recognition of presenting complaints and the ability to react effectively to life-threatening situations are all the domain of the triage practitioner

Table 3.2 (*Continued*)

Assessment component	Triage activity
	Focused questions can be used to obtain more detail if required, e.g. mechanism of injury, duration of the problem, current medications, etc. *The format of these questions will be directed by the discriminators in the chosen presentation flow chart*
Physical examination and assessment of physical parameters	If appropriate: • location of actual sites of injury • recording of baseline observations, pulse, temperature or more detailed information, e.g. obtained from pulse oximetry or assessment of visual acuity
Pain assessment	An integral part of the MTS, both subjective (patient) and objective (triage practitioner) pain scores are worth recording with documentation of the rationale for differing scores
Priority/plan of care	Priority assigned using the most appropriate discriminator applicable to the patient. Briefly describe any further care identified as a result of the triage assessment
Documentation	The recording of this information should be in an agreed format and should be clear, concise and relevant to the presenting complaint When a computerised triage system is in place, the triage practitioner should make sure the focus of attention is always the patient and not the computer screen/keyboard Include a record of any: • allergies • current medications • relevant past medical history • first aid measures applied at triage • observations • drugs administered, e.g. analgesia *Make sure signature is legible*
Reassessment	Document where there is a need to reassess, in particular when analgesia has been administered at triage

By following this systematic process, facilitated by the triage methodology, the patient assessment can be performed rapidly and confidently to reach an appropriate clinical priority in order to guide decision making.

Monitoring and evaluating

Clinical priority can change and triage must therefore be dynamic. The triage method described here can be carried out rapidly and reliably by qualified clinicians; it is therefore useful as a tool for multiple re-evaluations of clinical priority during the patient's stay.

Every encounter can be used as a triage assessment and any change in clinical priority can be rapidly notified and acted upon.

CHAPTER 4

Pain assessment as part of the triage process

Introduction

Pain is a key issue for patients attending Emergency Departments. Pain assessment has improved since the first edition of this text, however pain assessment must remain at the forefront of the triage method so that pain continues to be assessed and managed appropriately. Pain is an important issue for a number of reasons.

- The majority of patients attending Emergency Departments have some degree of pain
- The degree of pain influences the urgency
- The adequacy of pain management is a key criterion for patient satisfaction
- Patients in pain can become agitated and aggressive
- Patients in pain are a source of distress and stress to both staff and other patients
- Patients have an expectation that their pain will be dealt with

There are many advantages in assessing pain as part of the triage process. First, it ensures that a patient's pain is managed at the earliest opportunity – the provision of appropriate analgesia and consequent reduction in pain may lead to the possibility of re-categorisation to a lower priority. Patient anxiety is reduced and communication is improved. Without pain assessment the provision of appropriate analgesia at triage is not possible.

Emergency Triage: Manchester Triage Group, Third Edition.
Edited by Kevin Mackway-Jones, Janet Marsden and Jill Windle.
© 2014 John Wiley & Sons, Ltd. Published 2014 by John Wiley & Sons, Ltd.

Pain assessment at triage

Pain assessment is an integral part of the Manchester triage methodology. This is a deliberate and explicit recognition of the importance of pain and it is recognised that the result is that patients are categorised into a higher priority than was traditionally the case.

If a patient's pain is to be assessed formally at triage, and the outcome of that assessment is to help determine the urgency with which that patient is to be seen, then all triage practitioners must be competent in assessing pain, and the pain assessment must be valid and reproducible. It is unrealistic to expect that only the patient's subjective assessment will be taken into consideration during this process. By the same token it is inappropriate that the triage practitioners make their own subjective assessment of the patient's pain in isolation.

Pain assessment in the Emergency Department

This can be difficult because patients may be under pressure to say that their pain is severe so as to justify their attendance, and some patients, particularly children, may deny that they have pain to avoid having treatment or being admitted to hospital. Some practitioners' assessment and management of pain may be influenced by 'traditional' pathways of care. For example, patients who have fractures are offered immediate analgesia, but patients with abdominal pain may not be offered analgesia until the surgeons have seen them.

There may be concerns by staff that a patient will score pain higher if it is thought that this will result in a quicker treatment, but the objective assessment of pain will ameliorate this.

Pain assessment tools

Many Emergency Departments now use a formal pain assessment tool, but many such tools suffer from the fact that they were developed for use with postoperative and chronically ill patients.

There are three main types of pain assessment tools:

- Verbal descriptor scales
- Visual analogue scales
- Pain behaviour tools

Verbal descriptor scales

These scales consist of a number of word descriptors, usually three or five, which are numerically ranked. The most common descriptors are as follows:

- None
- Slight
- Moderate
- Severe
- Agonising

and the numerical value increases with the severity of the pain. The verbal descriptor scale is short and relatively easy for the patient to use and has been employed in the Emergency Department environment (Table 4.1).

Table 4.1

Advantages	Disadvantages
It provides a score which is easy for any practitioner to analyse	The use of a single word from a limited list may not reflect the pain that the patient is experiencing
It probably produces reliable data	It is not suitable for patients who do not speak English
It can be modified for use in children	It is the patient's subjective assessment

Visual analogue scales

These scales usually consist of a straight line representing varying levels of pain with verbal anchors at each end.

NO PAIN	PAIN AS BAD AS IT COULD BE

Patients can mark anywhere on the line. Verbal descriptors can also be added beneath the line in addition to the word anchors. The line can also be broken down to facilitate scoring for evaluation or comparative purposes.

Table 4.2

Advantages	Disadvantages
Easy and fast to use and score	Some patients choose to mark the line near one of the verbal anchors
These scales may be more sensitive than verbal descriptors	Certain patients find these scales too abstract to use, in particular those in severe pain, those with lower educational abilities or those with impaired motor coordination. The elderly can have some difficulty in using these scales
If used correctly they are reproducible and reliable	

Pain behaviour tools

These tools have been developed relying on the principle that patients who are in pain exhibit certain behaviours and physiological changes. These tools can measure the following:

- Verbal response
- Body language
- Facial expression
- Behavioural changes
- Conscious level
- Physiological changes

A number of different tools exist, each based on combining a number of the above factors, but have some disadvantages in use (Table 4.3).

Table 4.3

Advantages	Disadvantages
Can be used in patients with communication problems	Complex scales; comparison and scoring are difficult
	The patient's subjective assessment is not included
	Difficult to ensure that pain alone underlies the observed changes
	Time consuming, taking 5–15 minutes to use

The ideal pain assessment tool

An ideal tool for use in the Emergency Department should be simple and quick to use, should have been validated and must give reliable, reproducible results. These results should take account of both patient and observer data.

The pain ruler

No single pain assessment tool is better than another, although some would seem to be more suited to particular clinical areas than others. The pain ruler is a well-established pain assessment tool which would seem to lend itself for use in the Emergency Department setting more than some others. In particular, the advantages are as follows:

- It measures the intensity of pain and the effects on normal function
- It combines the use of verbal descriptors and a visual analogue scale
- It is fast and easy to use
- It is easily weighted to allow pain assessment to be part of the triage process
- By helping in the normal function assessment, the triage practitioner can become involved in the pain assessment process
- It promotes dialogue, which in turn encourages patients that their pain is being taken seriously
- It produces a score facilitating ongoing assessment
- The outcome of the assessment is quick and easy to document
- It can easily be adapted for use in children

A pain ruler offers scores of 0–10 but this is grouped into no pain, mild pain, moderate pain and severe pain, which is congruent with other pain scoring tools. These descriptions are used in the presentational flow charts. A pain ruler is shown in Figure 4.1.

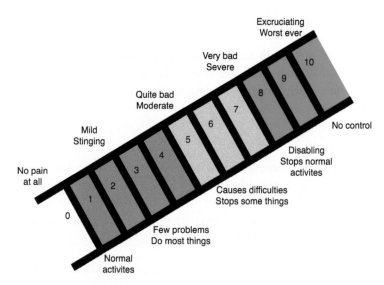

Figure 4.1 Pain ruler

This can be supplemented by a faces scale for use in small children as shown in Figure 4.2.

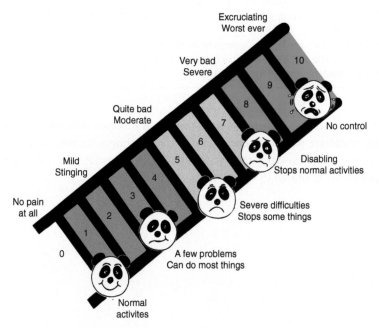

Figure 4.2 Faces scale pain ruler for use in smaller children

Pain assessment at triage

Pain assessment is a skilled process in any environment and the assessment carried out during triage is no exception. There are particular constraints in this setting reflecting the emergency nature of the patients and the lack of assessment time. Nevertheless, an accurate assessment of the patient's pain into one of the categories shown in the flow chart is essential if proper and timely care is to be given. The triage practitioner must take into account a number of factors that influence the patients' perception of their pain.

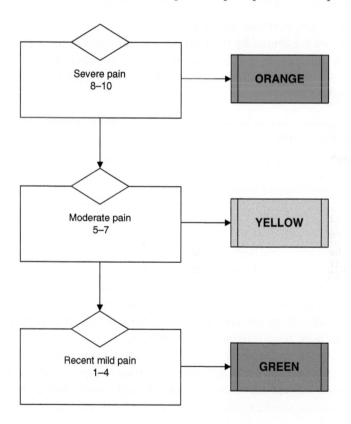

Age

Children may imagine the worst possible outcome of their pain. They use catastrophic thinking which increases their anxiety and fear and may therefore enhance their perception of pain. The practitioner must be able to recognise the signs of pain in pre-verbal children and the pain ruler can be adapted for this.

Many elderly people suffer from multiple pain problems and may consider a significant pain level to be normal. Many accept pain and cope well with it.

Assessment skill

- Recognise patients whose age affects pain assessment
- Is pain perception increased or decreased?
- How can this be overcome?

Previous experience of pain

Patients are influenced by their previous experiences of pain. They may compare this pain to previous episodes as to whether this is more or less severe. They will also be influenced by how the pain was managed previously.

Assessment skill

- Recognise whether the patient has had similar pain before
- What is different now?
- How did the patient manage the pain before?

Culture

Illness behaviour, and therefore pain behaviour, has a strong cultural component, and because of different cultural and social influences not all individuals express pain in the same way. Pain behaviour continues to be reinforced throughout life by the social group to which the individual belongs.

Particular cultural groups do not feel pain less than others, they only differ in how they respond to, or express, their pain. It is essential that the triage practitioners recognise that their own cultural and social background will inevitably influence how they interpret a patient's pain behaviour. This identifies one particular difficulty with relying on assessment tools that consider only the patient's (or the practitioner's) subjective assessment.

Assessment skill

- Recognise your own and the patient's cultural background
- How does this affect the patient's pain perception?
- How does this affect the observer's interpretation of behaviour?

Anxiety

There is a link between high anxiety levels and high pain scoring. Patients can be anxious for a number of reasons: they may be concerned about the effect of the illness/accident on their ability to carry out their everyday activities, and they may be anxious about attending hospital or worried about what is actually wrong with them.

There are considerable benefits in addressing a patient's pain at triage, in that the patient is shown at the earliest opportunity that his or her pain is being taken seriously. Reassurance and explanation from the triage practitioner at this time may play a part in effectively reducing the level of pain.

Assessment skill

- Recognise the level of anxiety of the patient
- What lies behind the patient's anxiety?
- How does this affect the patient's perception of pain?

Disruption to patient's usual activities

Any individual functions at a level which is what he, or she, considers to be normal. Pain can destroy the patient's ability to perform at that level, affecting their physical and emotional well-being, their financial situation and their position within society. Patients' perception of their pain will be influenced to some extent by how the pain will stop them functioning normally. It may not be possible to fully assess the level of disruption to the patient's usual activities, but the practitioner may be able to help the patient to focus on the effect of the pain by asking pertinent questions such as: Does the pain stop them eating/drinking/sleeping/breathing properly? Does the pain stop them walking/sitting? Does the pain stop them working/going to school?

Assessment skill

- Recognise the degree to which normal daily activities are disrupted
- How can the degree of disruption be assessed?
- How does the degree of disruption relate to the patient's perception of pain?

If a patient scores his pain as 10 but then is able to perform all his usual activities, the practitioner should consider other factors that may be influencing the patient's assessment of his pain.

Other considerations

Some patients may not be able to participate in the pain assessment process. They may be confused, have learning difficulties or be too distressed. Likewise, they may not be able to read or understand English. Consider each patient as an individual and think about other tools that you could use instead.

Assessment skill

- Recognise that no single assessment tool is appropriate for every patient presenting with pain
- Can this patient participate using this method of assessment?
- What other methods of pain assessment are more appropriate?

CHAPTER 5

Patient management, triage and the triage practitioner

Introduction

There is a difference between absolute clinical priority, as defined using the method in this book, and relative priority within and between triage categories. In overview, the process of triage, as outlined here, is quite simple – patients are assigned to a triage category and then managed in order of priority and time of attendance. However, there are many other factors apart from clinical priority which may, from time to time, influence how the patient is handled within the Emergency Department. This chapter outlines these factors and discusses their importance. Clinical priority and the findings that determine it are clearly very important, but failure to recognise other factors can be detrimental to both departmental function and quality of care for individual patients.

Type of patient

There are a number of issues about the nature of individual patients that affect their management in addition to their clinical priority. These are summarised below.

Children

Children may need specific consideration, especially in Emergency Departments without separate paediatric facilities. They are almost always accompanied by someone else (usually a parent – but teachers, relatives or social workers may also be present), as well as siblings and friends who, although well, need entertaining. Children have very short attention spans and get bored, frightened and tired very easily. They may become distressed and

---

Emergency Triage: Manchester Triage Group, Third Edition.
Edited by Kevin Mackway-Jones, Janet Marsden and Jill Windle.
© 2014 John Wiley & Sons, Ltd. Published 2014 by John Wiley & Sons, Ltd.

agitated because of communication and understanding difficulties, and this makes later handling more difficult.

Children who can be distracted by a play specialist, or in a separate waiting room with age-specific facilities, probably do not need any specific consideration other than frequent reassessment. It is helpful if child-friendly food and drink, e.g. snacks and drinks in cartons, bottles, etc., are available (provided the carer of any child who may need a general anaesthetic or sedation is aware of the need to keep the child nil by mouth).

It may be worthwhile having a policy for children who present late in the evening or at night. The child who is very tired may prove impossible to examine and treat, so a relatively early examination may be considered.

Elders
Relative immobility can cause increased discomfort in the waiting room and may cause difficulty for the patient in reaching the toilet or going for refreshments. A person who is normally able to cope well in familiar surroundings may become quite confused and disorientated in the Emergency Department. The elderly are very prone to pressure damage to tissues, which can develop after only half an hour on a hospital trolley. If they cannot be seen quickly for treatment, they need frequent nursing attention. They may have problems with continence which, if not anticipated, may lead to embarrassment. Cognitive difficulties may lead to them providing little information. Practitioners should be aware of these issues and consider the relative needs of this group of patients.

Patients with physical disability or learning difficulties
Apart from the extremes of age, there will be patients who have particular difficulties. These include those with special needs, poor sight, poor hearing, etc. Persons who can cope quite well in the community under controlled circumstances may have great difficulties in the strange environment of the Emergency Department. Communications again become particularly important, and it may be appropriate for such patients to be seen relatively quickly.

Abusive/aggressive patients
There are few things worse than having a full waiting room, with one or more patients (or more often relatives or friends of patients) constantly demanding attention. Although the guiding principle must be that these patients are not given priority just because they shout louder, the distress they cause to others must be taken into consideration. An initial

attempt to communicate departmental policy may be followed by a number of actions. The patient may be placed in an individual cubicle to wait in order to minimise the disruption to the waiting room. Alternatively, such patients can be seen, treated and discharged rapidly for the benefit of others. If all else fails, the patient (or the patient's relatives) may be asked to leave, assisted, as necessary, by security or the police.

Patients under the influence of alcohol

These patients are difficult to assess because of the effect of alcohol on conscious level and on pain perception. They need frequent reassessment to check that they are not deteriorating or developing a problem not immediately apparent at triage. Disruptive drunk patients should be managed as outlined above.

Frequent attenders

Most departments have a number of patients who are frequent attenders. It is undoubtedly tempting to place these patients in the non-urgent category without proper assessment. Beware, even this patient group develop organic pathology, injure themselves or have a serious complication of their disease. These patients (even those with predominantly social problems) are in fact more likely to develop illnesses or sustain injuries than the general population. Each attendance should be treated as a new visit and proper assessment should be undertaken; this avoids underestimation of possible serious causes for attending.

Patients who re-attend

There are occasions when patients return to the department, usually because their original presenting complaint has not resolved or they have developed a complication. Sometimes the patient's expectations of the natural progress of an injury or illness are unrealistic. The patient may also return having failed to wait for definitive treatment on a prior occasion. The patient should be allocated a triage category according to the symptoms presenting at the time of triage, and not according to the original triage category. Some departments may have policies recommending that such patients are reviewed by a senior doctor if available. It may also be appropriate to offer some of these patients a review clinic appointment for assessment by a senior doctor if the problem does not seem to need immediate treatment.

Clinic patients

Most Emergency Departments hold review clinics. Some services hold clinics in an area away from the department, and, although they may see Emergency Department staff, these patients would not impinge on the triage practitioner role. If the clinic is held within the Emergency Department, then it is usual for these patients to have a different priority and/or route through the department. It is important that the triage practitioner explains to the new patients that there are clinic patients who may be called out of turn.

Patients referred by other agencies

Many departments allow their facilities to be used by other teams for patient assessment. These patients are usually pre-arranged or accepted patients from primary care physicians. They are often patients who are accepted for possible admission and many have a relatively high clinical priority. *These patients must be triaged in the same way as Emergency Department patients.* If the patient is triaged as first priority it would be usual for the Emergency Department team to initiate resuscitation, unless the referral team is in the department. The triage practitioner should inform the referral team of the triage category of the patients in order to try and ensure that these patients are treated with a similar degree of urgency as Emergency Department patients. It may also be appropriate for the triage practitioner to ask departmental clinical staff to provide analgesia or initiate immediate investigations, in order to smooth the patients' stay in the department.

Some patients may have been brought in by the police (for instance under mental health legislation), by social services or by other professional services. Triage practitioners should be aware of the pressures on staff from other agencies and consider this when deciding on the management of such patients, but the triage priority would not change.

Departmental factors

Any department that deals with emergencies may at times be overwhelmed by the influx of patients. Sometimes, it only takes one seriously ill patient, or an absent member of staff, to produce a standstill. Each department needs to develop means of coping with this. An accurate triage assessment is an essential first step in good departmental management.

Both the workload and the staffing of the department will vary according to the time of day. Frequently overnight there is reduced clinical staffing. This may cause increased waiting times and difficulties in the waiting room, particularly if there are patients who are aggressive or under the influence of alcohol.

Fast tracking, streaming and matching resources to demand

Streaming is a term used to describe the splitting of patients into different groups who are then seen by staff dedicated to that particular group or stream. Once within a particular stream the patient is not affected by pressures elsewhere in the system. This is similar to the concept of 'fast tracking', where particular groups of patients (usually those with relatively minor injuries and illnesses) are identified and seen by dedicated staff to improve the flow. The main difference is that streaming is delivered as a planned intervention, rather than as a reactive one.

The Manchester Triage System can be used to facilitate streaming. This is discussed in detail in chapter 8.

Role of the triage practitioner

The triage practitioner's main role is the accurate prioritisation of patients and this must be the prime objective. The triage practitioner needs to become accomplished at rapid assessment – this involves quick decision making and suitable delegation of tasks. Long conversations with patients should be avoided, as should exhaustive history taking. Clinical observations, such as temperature/pulse, etc., need to be delegated if they are not required to establish priority as they are too time consuming.

In small departments, the triage practitioner will see all patients coming into the department. In others, there may be separate practitioners dealing with patients who arrive on foot or by ambulance. The mode of arrival of the patient does not always correlate with the seriousness of the presenting problem. (Patients with trivial complaints may call the emergency services and patients with a myocardial infarction may arrive by car.) Therefore there must be close liaison between triage and clinical areas to ensure that patients are placed in the appropriate location. The triage method outlined in this book should assist this process by standardising triage practice.

Rapid influxes of patients may require the triage practitioner to seek assistance from another member of staff. The triage process is integral to the clinical management of most departments, and a variety of additional tasks may be undertaken.

First aid/analgesia

The triage practitioner may need to provide or facilitate some first aid treatment, and recognise the need to provide analgesics if required (see chapter 4). Application of a sling or dressing will immediately improve the patient's comfort and help minimise further trauma and bleeding.

Patient information

The triage practitioner is the first clinical contact for the patient, and talking the patient through the illness and probable course in the department alleviates much distress and anxiety. Patients appreciate knowing the waiting time, the probable time spent in the department, whether any investigations may be ordered and possible treatment. This information can be provided quickly for most common conditions.

Health promotion

The triage practitioner (if time allows) can usefully act as a health promoter. The patient is usually quite receptive to health care advice when an adverse event has occurred. If possible brief advice about relevant topics, such as locked cabinets for medications, cycle helmets and smoking cessation, may be appropriate. It is helpful if patient information leaflets are available.

Disposition of patients around the department

The triage practitioner will often have to decide where to place the patients in the department. This will depend on departmental facilities and policies. Patients who are distressed, in pain, bleeding or at extremes of age may be best placed in cubicles away from the general waiting room. Patients who need to be lying down for examination (e.g. those suffering from knee injuries, back complaints and abdominal pain) should be placed in an area where they can lie down. Ill patients may well walk into the department and need to be placed in the appropriate area of the department. To achieve this, the triage practitioner needs to be continuously aware of the occupancy of the department and the current disposition of patients.

Managing the waiting room

Until they have been seen by a clinician, the patients' main contact is the triage practitioner. Further advice may be sought by these patients, and criticisms delivered. The triage practitioner needs to keep the occupants of the waiting room informed of the current approximate waiting time. Constant observation and reassessment are necessary in order to spot those patients whose condition is changing. Triage is a dynamic process and patients often need regular reassessment. This might occur after an intervention, e.g. the administration of analgesic, or after an appropriate length of time. Patients may be re-triaged into a lower category after pain relief or given higher priority if they deteriorate. No one can anticipate all problems and it is not a 'failure' of accurate assessment to change the triage category according to further developments in the patient's condition, or indeed with further information that may be acquired. The waiting room should be considered to be a clinical area and the domain and responsibility of the triage practitioner.

CHAPTER 6
Auditing the triage process

Introduction

When the Manchester Triage Group set out its aims at its very first meeting in November 1994, it clearly identified the need for a robust audit methodology. The reasons for this were, very simply, that the MTS was designed to reduce unwarranted variations in the triage process and this reduction could only be ensured by audit. Audit, in this context at least, is a quality management procedure; since triage is a fundamental cornerstone of clinical risk management, failure to ensure the quality of triage may have serious consequences.

Fortunately the Manchester Triage methodology is eminently auditable. The presentation–discriminator–priority progression (the process) by which individual triage practitioners arrive at their conclusions is easy for an auditor to note and easily assessable for accuracy by a trained assessor.

In addition to the process of triage discussed above, audit can also address other issues such as completeness of notes and adherence with terminology (it is not unusual for harassed triage practitioners to 'invent' a new discriminator if the actual discriminator has slipped their mind).

The aim of this chapter is to describe a robust triage audit method for the MTS and also to outline some of the results that have been found in audits around the world.

Audit method

At a basic level, the accuracy of individual triage practitioners underpins the whole quality agenda. Thus the most robust triage audit continuously assesses practitioners for accuracy and is linked by reflective practice and, if necessary, additional training to improved performance. The method outlined below is an audit of individual practitioner triage activity and is

Emergency Triage: Manchester Triage Group, Third Edition.
Edited by Kevin Mackway-Jones, Janet Marsden and Jill Windle.
© 2014 John Wiley & Sons, Ltd. Published 2014 by John Wiley & Sons, Ltd.

designed to audit the quality of decision making against the MTS standard, along with standards of record keeping and documentation.

- All triage practitioners are identified
- All episodes of triage are identified
- Episodes are all assigned to individual practitioners
- 2% of episodes per practitioner (minimum of 10 episodes) are randomly selected
- Episodes are assessed by a senior trained triage practitioner
- Completeness of episodes is expressed as a simple proportion
- Accuracy of episodes is expressed as a simple proportion
- Number of incomplete episodes is fed back to the practitioner
- Overall accuracy is fed back to the practitioner
- Any causes of inaccurate triage are fed back to the practitioner

---

To ensure consistency of audit, 10% of episodes assessed are performed independently by a second senior practitioner and any differences moderated by discussion. Continuous audit can be time consuming but is an excellent means of assessing standards of triage activity and decision making. A monthly audit is advised when MTS is introduced to a clinical area. Even in large departments triaging 100,000 patients each year, the number audited is only 2000 cases per year or 160 per month. The frequency of audit may be reduced to 3–6-monthly thereafter. The criteria in Table 6.1 have been shown to capture the essential components of a safe and reproducible triage system.

Table 6.1

Criteria	Yes	No	Comments
Correct use of presentational flow chart			
Specific discriminators correctly selected			*(record as seen on triage record)*
Pain score recorded			
Correct triage category assigned (based on patient presentation and discriminators)			
Demonstrated ability to navigate the computerised triage system			*(where applicable)*
Triage record legible and named			
Re-triaged where necessary			

Two important measures of the triage process are obtained: completeness and accuracy.

Completeness

An episode is complete if all the steps necessary to reach the conclusion have been undertaken. The method requires that the practitioner excludes *all* the discriminators in any higher priority. Thus if SpO_2 appears as a discriminator in the chart selected, then the episode would be incomplete if no result was recorded. The most common error is to fail to record a pain score.

Accuracy

An episode is recorded as accurate if both the presentation and discriminator selected are appropriate. It is important to realise that there may be appropriate alternatives (indeed the system is designed to ensure that this can occur); thus audit should be carried out by a practitioner with sufficient experience to make this judgment.

Targets

- 0% episodes incomplete
- 95% accuracy
- 95% agreement between assessors

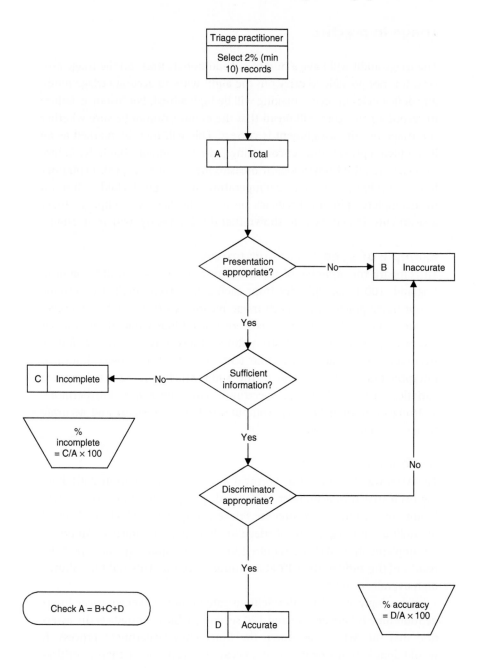

Triage in practice

The triage audit will have a number of additional effects on the triage process. It is not possible to carry out the audit without accurate triage notes; any deficiencies in record making will be highlighted. For instance, failure to record a pain score will mean that the auditor cannot be sure whether the triage priority assignment is correct. This will then be marked as an incomplete episode, thus encouraging pain assessment. Similarly, failure to record required physiological measurements, such as peak expiratory flow rate (PEFR) in asthma or temperature in the unwell child, will result in incomplete episodes. Feedback on a regular basis will improve these assessments. Experience has shown that this is an early 'win' from audit.

Example of a regional audit process

To compare the accuracy of the triage process across a health region in England, 100 triage episodes from each centre were audited by trained senior triage practitioners. Each triage record was reviewed by two practitioners and 10% of the records were triaged independently by further senior triage practitioners. A strong inter-observer agreement was found. Accuracy was found to vary from 68% to 95%. This allowed informed interpretation of the findings of the audit which demonstrated marked variation in case mix (triage spectrum) across the region. Furthermore, a strong association between computerised triage systems and accurate triage was demonstrated.

National triage audit

The MTS was introduced in Portugal as a national system in 2001 having been trialed in a number of hospitals prior to that time. The system is administered by the Portuguese Triage Group (GPT) which has insisted on audit as an integral part of triage in all its codes of practice. All hospitals implementing MTS are required to audit continuously and report the results of the audit to the GPT at an annual meeting. This audit has shown high overall accuracy.

Interestingly, audit has also demonstrated that the average triage intervention time is between 60 and 120 seconds, which contradicts the assertion that the MTS slows down the Emergency Department process. It would appear that slowing occurs because of tasks other than prioritisation carried out by triage practitioners as part of the initial assessment.

CHAPTER 7
Telephone triage

Introduction

The recognition of the need for formalised telephone triage and its development first occurred in the United States. Telephone triage was first described as a useful tool in the emergency setting in the United Kingdom in 1991. Various benefits have been attributed to this strategy including reduced attendance at the Emergency Department due to explanations and self-care advice, redirection of patients to more appropriate agencies, identification of problems before the patient attends the department, cost effectiveness and patient empowerment.

Giving advice by telephone has always been an integral part of the ED nurse's role although early studies suggested that patient assessment by telephone was subjective, poorly structured and carried out by untrained personnel. Decisions were made hastily without ascertaining the full facts. Recommendations arising from these studies were that a designated telephone advisor should be the first point of contact for telephone advice, protocols for informed advice for common problems should be developed and that adequate documentation was essential. Where these strategies have been implemented in practice, telephone assessment or triage has been found to be a safe and effective method of prioritisation. Formalised advice giving by telephone has the potential to be a valuable tool in many settings – a fact that was recognised in the development of national telephone advice helplines.

Telephone triage is distinct from telephone advice in that triage occurs when a formalised process of decision making takes place that allows

Emergency Triage: Manchester Triage Group, Third Edition.
Edited by Kevin Mackway-Jones, Janet Marsden and Jill Windle.
© 2014 John Wiley & Sons, Ltd. Published 2014 by John Wiley & Sons, Ltd.

identification of clinical priority, then allocation to predetermined categories of urgency of need for medical evaluation and care.

Telephone triage methodology

When undertaken effectively, triage involves a decision about clinical priority, which is based on presentation rather than diagnosis. Telephone triage should be undertaken in exactly the same way. The methodology described here builds on the effective face-to-face triage methodology taught by the Manchester Triage Group. The possible outcomes are, however, simplified from the five-category system as there are fewer options available to the telephone triage practitioner.

The decisions which must be made are as follows:

- Does the patient need immediate and urgent care? ('medicine now')
- Do they need care within the next few hours? ('medicine soon')
- Can medical or other care be delayed? ('medicine later')
- Advice only – where the problem can be managed by giving self-care advice

Patients who are in the 'medicine now' category are best served by the Emergency Ambulance Service and Emergency Departments, whatever the patients' locations. Those requiring 'medicine soon' or 'medicine later' may have care delivered in a number of locations and by various providers. Thus, the time to care in the 'medicine soon' category will vary, depending upon those services available in that health economy. A mapping exercise should be undertaken locally to agree the appropriate dispositions arising from the triage decision (see chapter 8). It is essential that the practitioner undertaking telephone triage uses up-to-date details about current local services, such as dental emergency arrangements, telephone numbers of primary care facilities and the location of all-night pharmacies.

Making the decision

On receiving the telephone call, the practitioner must gather some basic information from the caller about the nature of the problem. This will dictate which presentational flow chart is selected.

Once the decision has been made, questioning techniques are used to elicit information in order to decide what priority should be allocated. The methodology is reductive – working from more serious to less serious discriminators, and the triage practitioner is prompted to cover all possibilities by the information contained on the flow charts.

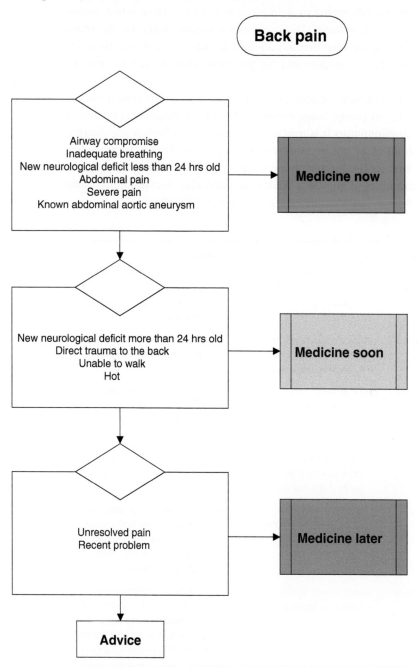

The practitioner must decide whether the criteria for each discriminator are fulfilled, and which of the discriminators present leads to the highest clinical priority. Discriminator definitions remain the same when undertaking triage by telephone. The questions normally asked by the triage practitioner must be modified to take into account the remoteness of the patient, the levels of anxiety and the possibility that the caller is not the patient.

Some discriminators appear in the face-to-face charts which do not appear in the telephone triage edition of *Emergency Triage*. This is because for some discriminators it is impossible to ascertain whether the discriminator is fulfilled or not without seeing the patient. Those discriminators are therefore not used in telephone triage.

Some examples of questions relating to particular discriminators, along with the discriminator definitions, are shown in Table 7.1.

Table 7.1

Discriminator	Questions	Definition
Acute onset after injury	Did this start after you fell/were hit, etc.? When did this start?	Onset of symptoms immediately or shortly after a recent physically traumatic event
Acutely avulsed tooth	When did your tooth come out? Was this the result of injury? Is it complete with a root?	A tooth that has been avulsed intact within the previous 24 hours
Acutely short of breath	Have you suddenly become short of breath? Are you more short of breath than normal?	Shortness of breath that comes on suddenly, or a sudden exacerbation of chronic shortness of breath
Altered conscious level	Do they open their eyes or move when you speak to them or gently shake their shoulders?	Not fully alert. Either responding to voice or pain only or unresponsive
Cardiac pain	Where is the pain? Have you had pain like this before? What is it like? Does it go to your arm or neck?	Classically a severe dull 'gripping' or 'heavy' pain in the centre of the chest, radiating to the left arm or to the neck. May be associated with sweating and nausea
Direct trauma to the neck	Have you been hit on your neck? What exactly happened?	This may be top to bottom (loading) for instance when something falls on the head, bending (forwards, backwards or to the side), twisting or distracting such as in hanging

Table 7.1 (*Continued*)

Discriminator	Questions	Definition
High risk of self-harm	What are you (they) going to do? Do you want to kill yourself?	An initial view of the risk of self-harm can be formed by considering the patient's behaviour. Patients who have a significant history of self-harm, who are actively trying to harm themselves or who are actively trying to leave with the intent of harming themselves are at high risk
Inconsolable by parent	Can you calm them down at all? Do they settle at all when you cuddle them?	Children whose crying or distress does not respond to attempts by their parents to comfort them fulfill this criteria
Signs of dehydration	Do you (they) have a dry tongue? Do you (they) look dry? Are you (they) passing as much urine as normal?	These include: dry tongue, sunken eyes, decreased skin turgor and, in small babies, a sunken anterior fontanelle. Usually associated with a low urine output
Signs of meningism	Do you (they) have a stiff neck? Does the light hurt your (their) eyes?	Classically a stiff neck together with headache and photophobia

Interim advice

Because the patient is remote from the triage practitioner, interim advice may be necessary in order to promote recovery or prevent deterioration in the condition of the patient before medical help is accessed. For example, if the triage practitioner obtains information that the patient is not breathing properly or has a compromised airway, then life-saving basic life support advice must be given to the caller so that resuscitation can be attempted until help arrives. Similarly if a child is unwell and is triaged to 'medicine later', it may be appropriate to give the carer advice on simple measures to alleviate symptoms such as fever and diarrhoea. Interim advice should be available for each discriminator. Some examples are shown in Table 7.2.

Table 7.2

Discriminator	Interim advice
Currently fitting	Attempt to place the patient in a recovery position (describe if necessary). Loosen clothing. Do not attempt to place anything into the mouth
History of overdose or poisoning	Do not try to induce vomiting. If lips are burning after ingestion of a corrosive substance try frequent sips of cold water
Hot child	Remove warm clothing. Administer paracetamol elixir if available, dosing according to the manufacturer's recommendations
Open fracture	Do not move the limb. Place pads or cushions around it to keep it still. Cover the wound with a clean pad or towel

Once details of the patient's presenting symptoms have been obtained, a priority category allocated and any appropriate interim advice given, then advice on transport may be necessary. Protocols for this may be agreed locally, depending on the telephone triage setting. Advice must also be given about what to do should the condition or circumstances of the patient change in the interim.

Pain

Pain assessment is an integral part of the triage decision-making process but presents special problems in a telephone triage situation. Not only is observation impossible, but the time taken to elicit specific information about pain may be limited and the patient or carer's understanding of what the triage practitioner means when asked about pain scales may be suboptimal.

The pain evaluation tool within the telephone triage system has been modified to reflect these difficulties. Severe pain is used as a discriminator to prioritise the patient into the 'medicine now' category in all cases. Severe pain warrants urgent investigation and management. Pain does not feature in any other decisions about clinical priority, which must be made on the basis of other information gained by the practitioner.

The telephone triage practitioner

Telephone triage, like face-to-face triage, should be undertaken by experienced practitioners. The availability of protocols and charts does not remove the need for expert clinical knowledge. Arguably the decisions made in telephone triage call for a higher level of skill and knowledge than when the patient is present. Furthermore, the questioning skills of the practitioner must be very highly developed in order to obtain the most useful information from a troubled caller in the least possible time.

Like face-to-face triage, telephone triage works well when it is carried out correctly and less well when arbitrary decisions are made, or important aspects such as pain are ignored. Systems must be auditable and this relies on good training of competent practitioners using their skills and knowledge and the tools available to them to the best effect.

The telephone triage methodology provides an effective and auditable tool for the prioritisation of patients presenting to immediate care settings by telephone.

CHAPTER 8

Beyond prioritisation

The Manchester Triage System was designed to be a robust, auditable clinical risk management tool that identified the clinical priority of individual patients. However, as has been mentioned earlier in this book, the process itself and the outcome of the process can also be useful beyond prioritisation. Two such uses are described here.

Monitoring of physiological parameters

Triage is a dynamic process and should be undertaken periodically on all patients while they are waiting for treatment. In this way any change in status can be identified and the triage category can be modified if necessary. The need for monitoring does not stop after first clinician contact – it is very important that any deterioration is identified as soon as possible so that appropriate reassessment can be undertaken and any treatments started. The similarity between post triage monitoring (dynamic triage) and post clinical assessment monitoring is self-evident.

In some areas of the hospital, ongoing monitoring uses an 'early warning score' format very successfully. In the Emergency Department, however, this may require clinicians to learn and implement a new assessment tool. The discriminators within the MTS, particularly those addressing ABCD life threat, lend themselves well to ongoing assessment and can easily be adapted into an early warning tool (Table 8.1). The use of these MTS-based physiological parameters ensures Emergency Department clinicians are familiar with this process and can quickly identify deterioration (or improvement) in the patient's condition that might need intervention.

Emergency Triage: Manchester Triage Group, Third Edition.
Edited by Kevin Mackway-Jones, Janet Marsden and Jill Windle.
© 2014 John Wiley & Sons, Ltd. Published 2014 by John Wiley & Sons, Ltd.

Table 8.1

	Red	Orange	Yellow
Airway	Airway compromise		
Breathing	Inadequate breathing	Very low SpO$_2$ Acutely short of breath	Low SpO$_2$

Circulation	Shock
	Exsanguinating
	   haemorrhage
		Abnormal pulse
		Marked tachycardia
		Uncontrollable major
		   haemorrhage
			Uncontrollable minor
			   haemorrhage

Disability	Unresponsive child Hypoglycaemia	Altered conscious level	

As with all monitoring tools, it is change rather than absolute score that is important. Thus the new appearance of a red discriminator should indicate immediate clinical reassessment, while the recognition of an orange or yellow discriminator should precipitate clinical action within 10 or 60 minutes, respectively. This approach has the advantage of using a tool with which the nursing staff are familiar, within a framework that is also well known.

Other uses of the triage consultation

Often the triage event includes more than the assessment and prioritisation of patients. In addition to being asked to prioritise patients and deliver basic first aid, practitioners may also be expected to do the following:
- Administer analgesia
- Refer patients directly for radiological investigations – in particular those with upper and lower limb injuries
- Triage patients to self-care, pharmacy services, GP non-urgent appointments or Out of Hours Service
- Initiate agreed patient pathways to facilitate direct referral to inpatient specialties

In many cases these activities will require a higher level of decision making than has previously been expected. There will be some associated training needs in the assessment of patients and understanding of the referral process in order for the clinician to make the choice of service that best meets the patient's needs.

The benefits of 'value added' or extended triage are that patients have access to pain management at the point of entry, where a delay in definitive treatment may be encountered. There is likely to be a reduction in the total time spent in the department if patients present to the treating clinician with radiographs ready for interpretation. Patients may avoid unnecessary delay if directed to alternative services/specialties from triage.

The downside to this approach is obvious; introducing more intervention in the assessment will result in longer consultation times and may create a significant delay for patients entering the system, thus introducing an element of risk. To offset this problem it is feasible to have more than one triage practitioner operating at any given time to ensure all patients are triaged without significant delay. As previously noted, the time needed for accurate prioritisation is only 60–120 seconds and it is therefore disingenuous to blame the triage event itself for any delays that result from widening the remit of initial assessment.

Presentation–priority matrix mapping

As the idea of the inappropriate patient becomes replaced by the concepts of inappropriate care delivery and patient choice, multiple entry gates to emergency care and the 'emergency care village' become realities. Clinicians must be equipped with tools that enable them to decide safely and effectively where patients might be best managed.

It became clear while reviewing the second edition of *Emergency Triage* that the outcome of the prioritisation process could be captured to inform decisions about the most appropriate disposition of the patient. In particular the combination of the presentational chart used and the priority allocated (the presentation–priority matrix, PPM) could be matched to particular types of emergency care provision. Thus a patient presenting with a limb problem and allocated to the green/4/standard priority should be seen in the Minor Treatment Area, while a patient with chest pain allocated to the orange/2/very urgent priority is best managed in the Resuscitation Room.

The MTS consists of 53 presentations most with five priorities – making a total of 258 presentation–priority combinations. A mapping exercise should be undertaken to consider appropriate dispositions for each of these priority presentations. The dispositions available will be subject to local emergency care provision, for example the lack of an Emergency Eye Unit will change where patients with eye problems are managed. An identified lack of a service may stimulate debate with the local commissioners in order to provide a more appropriate service for patients.

Explanation of the process

When making decisions as to the most appropriate disposition for patients it is important to identify a range of stakeholders who will work to develop the matrix, finally reaching a consensus decision. Where patients will be directed across a range of services it is useful to engage different providers and different professionals to give a balanced view of how patients will be directed.

Completing the PPM

- Establish the list of dispositions to which patients can be directed (see examples below)
- Provide each stakeholder with a blank matrix and a copy of the 3rd edition of *Emergency Triage*; this is strictly an open book exercise to ensure each stakeholder bases their decisions on the same methodology the triage practitioners will be using
- The stakeholders should individually use a reductionist approach (start at priority 1/red and work along the priorities to priority 5/blue) to consider for each of the presentation charts which disposition is appropriate for the patient in a particular priority, for example:

  Unwell adult – priority 1 – inadequate breathing = Resuscitation Room
  Dental problems – priority 4 – recent mild pain = Dental Service
  Limb problem – priority 3 – moderate pain = Minor Treatment Area

- All completed matrices should be collated; where consensus is not reached further iteration is required until a clear map of agreed dispositions is produced
- This process can and should be repeated at intervals to ensure any change in services is represented in the matrix

The dispositions

This example illustrates an agreed list for an emergency service that forms the basis of dispositions within the presentation–priority matrix (Table 8.2). Triage practitioners use the matrix to inform their decisions of where to best place a patient within that system. The triage practitioner will need to exercise judgment as to which is the most appropriate, as the decision may also be influenced by the availability of services across the

Table 8.2 Presentation–priority matrix 2011

	1	2	3	4	5
Abdominal pain in adults	R	Ma	Ma	PC	PC
Abdominal pain in children	R	R/Ma	Ma	PC	PC
Abscesses and local infection	R	Ma	Mi	PC	PC
Abuse and neglect	R	R	Ma	Mi	
Allergy	R	R	Ma	PC	PC
Apparently drunk	R	R/Ma	Ma	Mi	SC
Assault	R	R	Ma	Mi	SC
Asthma	R	R	Ma	PC	PC
Back pain	R	Ma	Mi	PC	PC
Behaving strangely	R	Ma	Mi/PSY	Mi/PSY	
Bites and stings	R	R	Mi	PC	PC
Burns and scalds	R	R	Ma	Mi	SC
Chemical exposure	R	R	Ma	Mi	PC
Chest pain	R	R	Ma	Mi	PC
Collapse	R	R	Ma	Mi	PC
Crying baby	R	R	Ma	PC	PC
Dental problems	R	Ma	Mi	Dent	Dent
Diabetes	R	R/Ma	Ma	PC	PC
Diarrhoea and vomiting	R	R	Ma	PC	SC
Ear problems	R	Ma	Ma	PC	PC
Eye problems	Ma	Ma	Mi/eye	Mi	PC
Facial problems	R	R/Ma	Ma	Mi	PC
Falls	R	R/Ma	Ma	Mi	PC
Fits	R	R	Ma	Mi	PC
Foreign body	R	R/Ma	Mi	Mi	PC
GI bleeding	R	R	Ma	PC	PC

Table 8.2 (*Continued*)

	1	2	3	4	5
Headache	R	R	Ma	Mi	PC
Head injury	R	R	Ma	Mi	SC
Irritable child	R	R	Ma	PC	PC
Limb problems	R	R	Ma	Mi	PC
Limping child	R	R	Ma	Mi	PC
Major trauma	R	R	Ma		
Mental illness	R	Ma	PSY	PSY	
Neck pain	R	Ma	Mi	PC	SC
Overdose and poisoning	R	Ma	Ma	Mi	
Palpitations	R	R	Ma	PC	PC
Pregnancy	R	R	Ma	PC	PC
PV bleeding	R	R/Ma	Ma	PC	PC
Rashes	R	R	Mi	PC	SC
Self-harm	R	R	Mi/PSY	Mi/PSY	
Sexually acquired infection	R	R/Ma	Mi	PC	SC
Shortness of breath in adults	R	R	Ma	PC	PC
Shortness of breath in children	R	R	Ma	PC	PC
Sore throat	R	Ma	Mi	PC	SC
Testicular pain	R	Ma	Mi	Mi	PC
Torso injury	R	R	Mi	Mi	PC
Unwell adult	R	R	Ma	PC	PC
Unwell baby	R	R	Ma	Mi	Mi
Unwell child	R	R	Ma	PC	PC
Unwell newborn	R	R	Ma	Mi	Mi
Urinary problems	R	Ma	Ma	PC	PC
Worried parent	R	R	Ma	PC	PC
Wounds	R	R/Ma	Mi	Mi	SC

24 hours, the current pressures on them, the triage discriminator and the patients' choices.

Triage disposition code	Disposition description
R	Resuscitation Room
Ma	Major Treatment Area
Mi	Minor Treatment Area
PC	Primary Care
SC	Self-care
PHAR	Pharmacy
PSY	Psychiatric Assessment/Crisis Team
DENT	Dental Service
SHC	Sexual Health Clinic
EYE	Eye Hospital or Clinic

It is apparent that Mi and PC dispositions are professionally led rather than patient led. It would be possible to provide both these services within a single area – perhaps an 'Urgent Care Centre' or 'Rapid Assessment and Treatment Unit', both of which approximately map onto the current 'minor end' of many Emergency Departments. There is obvious potential for many of these emergency/urgent care services to coalesce within an 'emergency care village' that also offers out of hours primary care provision.

The psychiatric disposition will be provided differently throughout the world and may include psychiatry and psychiatric nursing. Many Emergency Departments have Emergency Psychiatric Nursing Teams and some are developing Psychiatric Assessment Unit functions.

Emergency Dental Service and Eye Emergency Clinic dispositions will depend on local provision. The Sexual Health Clinic disposition will again depend on location and opening times of local provision, although the specialist nature of the care delivered will dictate that most patients not requiring immediate or very urgent care are redirected. Other dispositions may be available locally and should be used where appropriate, however, the decision will also depend on opening times and the location of any such facilities. There may be a tendency to place more than one disposition against a priority. Where services are not 24/7, or two or more services are acceptable and patients can make a choice, the triage practitioner will exercise judgment as to which is the most appropriate.

Black boxes in Table 8.2 indicate that the MTS does not have the presentation–priority outcome indicated by the box, e.g. mental illness does not have a priority 5 (blue) in the system.

This 'pigeon holing' can be used to drive pathways of care in systems that have taken to 'streaming'. Particular presentation–priority combinations (e.g. wounds–green, chest pain–orange) may be appropriate to particular streams (minor injuries and resuscitation, respectively, in the examples given). An unpopulated priority matrix is included on each of the presentational flow charts in order to stimulate discussion around context-specific dispositions.

Future uses

The MTS has undoubtedly been used to assist in other processes within hospital and pre-hospital practice. Whenever any uses beyond prioritisation are considered it should always be remembered that the system was designed to prioritise Emergency Department patients and any utility in processes other than this must be proved rather than assumed.

Presentational flow chart index

Emergency Triage: Manchester Triage Group, Third Edition.
Edited by Kevin Mackway-Jones, Janet Marsden and Jill Windle.
© 2014 John Wiley & Sons, Ltd. Published 2014 by John Wiley & Sons, Ltd.

Presentation	Pages
Head injury	118
Irritable child	120
Limb problems	122
Limping child	124
Major trauma	126
Mental illness	128
Neck pain	130
Overdose and poisoning	132
Palpitations	134
Pregnancy	136
PV bleeding	138
Rashes	140
Self-harm	142
Sexually acquired infection	144
Shortness of breath in adults	146
Shortness of breath in children	148
Sore throat	150
Testicular pain	152
Torso injury	154
Unwell adult	156
Unwell baby	158
Unwell child	160
Unwell newborn	162
Urinary problems	164
Worried parent	166
Wounds	168
Major incident – primary	170
Major incident – secondary	172

Presentational flow charts

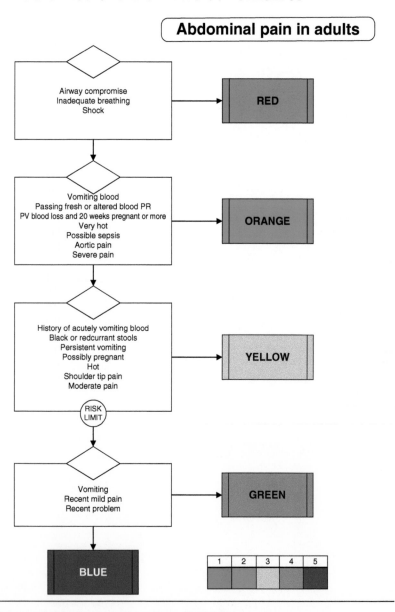

Abdominal pain in adults

Airway compromise
Inadequate breathing
Shock

RED

Vomiting blood
Passing fresh or altered blood PR
PV blood loss and 20 weeks pregnant or more
Very hot
Possible sepsis
Aortic pain
Severe pain

ORANGE

History of acutely vomiting blood
Black or redcurrant stools
Persistent vomiting
Possibly pregnant
Hot
Shoulder tip pain
Moderate pain

YELLOW

RISK
LIMIT

Vomiting
Recent mild pain
Recent problem

GREEN

BLUE

1	2	3	4	5

Emergency Triage: Manchester Triage Group, Third Edition.
Edited by Kevin Mackway-Jones, Janet Marsden and Jill Windle.
© 2014 John Wiley & Sons, Ltd. Published 2014 by John Wiley & Sons, Ltd.

Notes accompanying abdominal pain in adults

See also	Chart notes
Diarrhoea and vomiting GI bleeding Pregnancy	This is a presentation defined flow diagram. Abdominal pain is a common cause of presentation of surgical emergencies. A number of general discriminators are used including *Life threat* and *Pain*. Specific discriminators are included in the ORANGE and YELLOW categories to ensure that the more severe pathologies are appropriately triaged. In particular, discriminators are included to ensure that patients with moderate and severe GI bleeding and those with signs of retroperitoneal or diaphragmatic irritation are given sufficiently high categorisation

Specific discriminators	Explanation
Vomiting blood	Vomited blood may be fresh (bright or dark red) or coffee ground in appearance
Passing fresh or altered blood PR	In active massive GI bleeding dark red blood will be passed per rectum (PR). As GI transit time increases this becomes darker, eventually becoming melaena
PV blood loss and 20 weeks pregnant or more	Any loss of blood PV in a woman known to be beyond the 20th week of pregnancy
Possible sepsis	Suspected sepsis in patients who present with altered mental state, low blood pressure (systolic less than 100) or raised respiratory rate (rate more than 22). In children, age specific physiological tools should be used to determine if possibly septic
Aortic pain	The onset of symptoms is sudden and the leading symptom is severe abdominal or chest pain. The pain may be described as sharp, stabbing or ripping in character. Classically aortic chest pain is felt around the sternum and then radiates to the shoulder blades, aortic abdominal pain is felt in the centre of the abdomen and radiates to the back. The pain may get better or even vanish and then recur elsewhere. Over time, pain may also be felt in the arms, neck, lower jaw, stomach or hips
History of acutely vomiting blood	Frank haematemesis, vomiting of altered blood (coffee ground) or of blood mixed in the vomit within the past 24 hours
Black or redcurrant stools	Any blackness fulfils the criteria of black stool while a dark red stool, classically seen in intussusceptions, is redcurrant stool
Persistent vomiting	Vomiting that is continuous or that occurs without any respite between episodes
Possibly pregnant	Any woman whose normal menstruation has failed to occur is possibly pregnant. Furthermore any woman of childbearing age who is having unprotected sex should be considered to be potentially pregnant
Shoulder tip pain	Pain felt in the tip of the shoulder. This often indicates diaphragmatic irritation
Vomiting	Any emesis

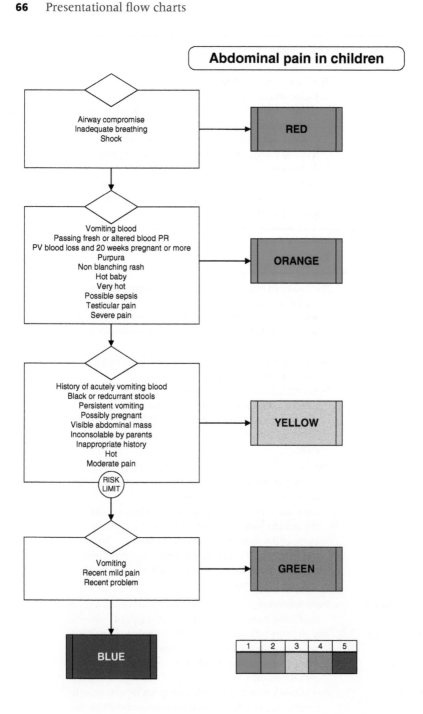

Abdominal pain in children

Airway compromise
Inadequate breathing
Shock

RED

Vomiting blood
Passing fresh or altered blood PR
PV blood loss and 20 weeks pregnant or more
Purpura
Non blanching rash
Hot baby
Very hot
Possible sepsis
Testicular pain
Severe pain

ORANGE

History of acutely vomiting blood
Black or redcurrant stools
Persistent vomiting
Possibly pregnant
Visible abdominal mass
Inconsolable by parents
Inappropriate history
Hot
Moderate pain

RISK
LIMIT

YELLOW

Vomiting
Recent mild pain
Recent problem

GREEN

BLUE

| 1 | 2 | 3 | 4 | 5 |

Notes accompanying abdominal pain in children

See also	Chart notes
Diarrhoea and vomiting Unwell newborn	This is a presentation defined flow diagram. Children who present with abdominal pain may have a range of pathologies and this chart has been designed to allow them to be accurately prioritised. A number of general discriminators are used including *Life threat* and *Pain*. Specific discriminators are included to ensure the children who are actively bleeding, and those who have the signs or symptoms of more severe pathologies such as intussusception, are seen urgently. If the patient is under 28 days, the Unwell Newborn chart should be used

Specific discriminators	Explanation
Vomiting blood	Vomited blood may be fresh (bright or dark red) or coffee ground in appearance
Passing fresh or altered blood PR	In active massive GI bleeding dark red blood will be passed PR. As GI transit time increases this becomes darker, eventually becoming melaena
PV blood loss and 20 weeks pregnant or more	Any loss of blood PV in a woman known to be beyond the 20th week of pregnancy
Purpura	A rash on any part of the body that is caused by small haemorrhages under the skin. A purpuric rash does not blanch (go white) when pressure is applied to it
Non-blanching rash	A rash that does not blanch (go white) when pressure is applied to it. Often tested using a glass tumbler to apply pressure as any colour change can be observed through the bottom of the tumbler
Signs of severe pain	Young children and babies in severe pain cannot complain. They will usually cry out continuously and inconsolably and be tachycardic. They may well exhibit signs such as pallor and sweating
Possible sepsis	Suspected sepsis in patients who present with altered mental state, low blood pressure (systolic less than 100) or raised respiratory rate (rate more than 22). In children, age specific physiological tools should be used to determine if possibly septic
Testicular pain	Pain in the testicles
History of acutely vomiting blood	Frank haematemesis, vomiting of altered blood (coffee ground) or of blood mixed in the vomit within the past 24 hours
Black or redcurrant stools	Any blackness fulfils the criteria of black stool while a dark red stool, classically seen in intussusceptions, is redcurrant stool
Persistent vomiting	Vomiting that is continuous or that occurs without any respite between episodes
Possibly pregnant	Any woman whose normal menstruation has failed to occur is possibly pregnant. Furthermore any woman of childbearing age who is having unprotected sex should be considered to be potentially pregnant
Visible abdominal mass	A mass in the abdomen that is visible to the naked eye
Inconsolable by parents	Children whose crying or distress does not respond to attempts by their parents to comfort them
Inappropriate history	When the history (story) given does not explain the physical findings it is termed inappropriate. This is important as it is a marker of safeguarding concerns in both adults and children
Vomiting	Any emesis

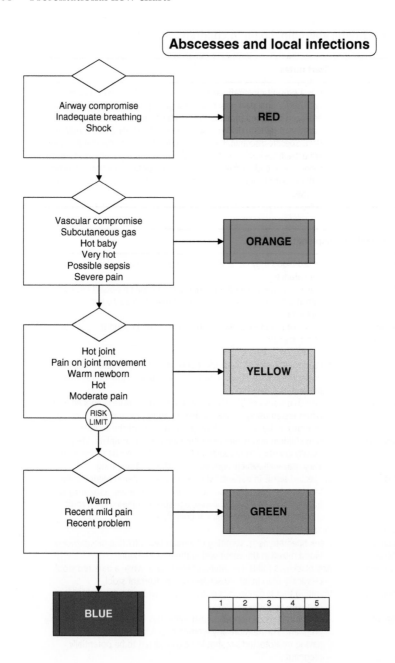

Abscesses and local infections

Airway compromise	**RED**
Inadequate breathing	
Shock	

Vascular compromise	**ORANGE**
Subcutaneous gas	
Hot baby	
Very hot	
Possible sepsis	
Severe pain	

Hot joint	**YELLOW**
Pain on joint movement	
Warm newborn	
Hot	
Moderate pain	

RISK LIMIT

Warm	**GREEN**
Recent mild pain	
Recent problem	

BLUE

1	2	3	4	5

Notes accompanying abscesses and local infections

See also	Chart notes
Bites and stings	This is a presentation defined flow diagram designed to allow prioritisation of patients who present with a variety of obvious local infections and abscesses. Underlying conditions may vary from life-threatening orbital cellulitis to acneiform spots. A number of general discriminators are used including *Life threat*, *Pain* and *Temperature*. Specific discriminators have been included to allow identification of more urgent conditions such as gas gangrene and septic arthritis

Specific discriminators	Explanation
Vascular compromise	There will be a combination of pallor, coldness, altered sensation and pain with or without absent pulses distal to the injury
Subcutaneous gas	Gas under the skin can be detected by feeling for a 'crackling' on touch. There may be gas bubbles and a line of demarcation
Possible sepsis	Suspected sepsis in patients who present with altered mental state, low blood pressure (systolic less than 100) or raised respiratory rate (rate more than 22). In children, age specific physiological tools should be used to determine if possibly septic
Hot joint	Any warmth around a joint. Often accompanied by redness
Pain on joint movement	This can be pain on either active (patient) movement or passive (examiner) movement

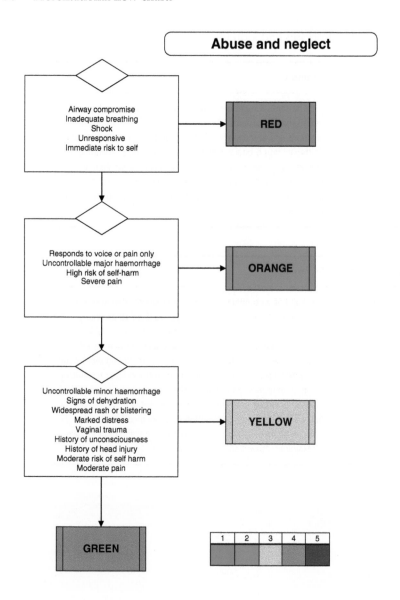

Notes accompanying Abuse and neglect

See also	Chart notes
	This is a presentation defined flow diagram designed to allow prioritisation of patients who present with signs of abuse or neglect. This chart is not designed to triage illness or injury but rather to triage children whose presentation is abuse or neglect. If the presentation is physical illness or injury, it would be more appropriate to use different charts. A number of general discriminators are used including *Life threat*, *Conscious level* and *Pain*. Specific discriminators have been included to allow prioritisation of the most urgent cases

Specific discriminators	Explanation
Unresponsive	Patients who fail to respond to either verbal or painful stimuli
Responds to voice or pain only	Responds to a vocal or painful stimulus
High risk of self-harm	An initial view of the risk of harm to self can be formed by considering the patient's behaviour. Patients who are threatening to harm themselves and who are actively seeking the means to do so are at high risk
Signs of dehydration	These include dry tongue, sunken eyes, decreased skin turgor and, in small babies, a sunken anterior fontanelle. Usually associated with a low urine output
Widespread rash or blistering	Any discharging or blistering eruption covering more than 10% of the body surface area
Marked distress	Patients who are markedly physically or emotionally upset
Vaginal trauma	Any history or other evidence of direct trauma to the vagina
History of head injury	A history of a recent physically traumatic event involving the head. Usually this will be reported by the patient but if the patient has been unconscious this history should be sought from a reliable witness
Moderate risk of self harm	An initial view of the risk of harm to self can be formed by considering the patient's behaviour. Patients without a significant history of self harm, who are not actively trying to harm themselves, but who profess the desire to harm themselves are at moderate risk

Allergy

Airway compromise
Stridor
Drooling
Inadequate breathing
Shock
Unresponsive child

→ RED

Oedema of the tongue
Facial oedema
Unable to talk in sentences
Very low SpO$_2$
New abnormal pulse
Altered conscious level
Significant history of allergy
Severe pain or itch

→ ORANGE

Low SpO$_2$
Widespread rash or blistering
Moderate pain or itch

→ YELLOW

RISK LIMIT

Local inflammation
Recent mild pain or itch
Recent problem

→ GREEN

BLUE

1	2	3	4	5

Notes accompanying allergy

See also	Chart notes
Asthma Bites and stings Collapse Unwell adult	This is a presentation defined flow diagram designed to allow prioritisation of patients who present with symptoms and signs that may indicate allergy. Patients with allergic reactions range from those with life-threatening anaphylaxis to those with an itchy insect bite. A number of general discriminators are used including *Life threat*, *Conscious level* and *Pain*. Specific discriminators have been included to allow prioritisation of the most urgent conditions

Specific discriminators	Explanation
Stridor	This may be an inspiratory or expiratory noise, or both. Stridor is heard best on breathing with the mouth open
Drooling	Saliva running from the mouth as a result of being unable to swallow
Oedema of the tongue	Swelling of the tongue of any degree
Facial oedema	Diffuse swelling around the face, usually involving the lips
Unable to talk in sentences	Patients who are so breathless that they cannot complete relatively short sentences in one breath
Very low SpO$_2$	This is a saturation of less than 95% on O$_2$ therapy or less than 92% on air
New abnormal pulse	A bradycardia (less than 60/min in adults), a tachycardia (more than 100/min in adults) or an irregular rhythm. Age-appropriate definitions of bradycardia and tachycardia should be used in children
Significant history of allergy	A known sensitivity with severe reaction (e.g. to nuts or bee sting) is significant
Low SpO$_2$	This is a saturation of less than 95% on air
Widespread rash or blistering	Any discharging or blistering eruption covering more than 10% of the body surface area
Local inflammation	Local inflammation will involve pain, swelling and redness confined to a particular site or area

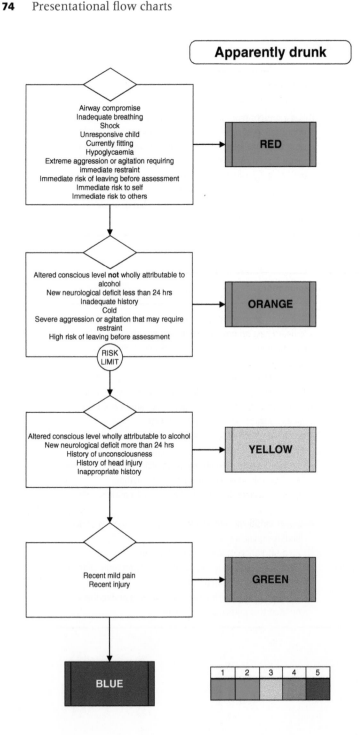

Apparently drunk

Airway compromise
Inadequate breathing
Shock
Unresponsive child
Currently fitting
Hypoglycaemia
Extreme aggression or agitation requiring immediate restraint
Immediate risk of leaving before assessment
Immediate risk to self
Immediate risk to others

RED

Altered conscious level **not** wholly attributable to alcohol
New neurological deficit less than 24 hrs
Inadequate history
Cold
Severe aggression or agitation that may require restraint
High risk of leaving before assessment

ORANGE

RISK LIMIT

Altered conscious level wholly attributable to alcohol
New neurological deficit more than 24 hrs
History of unconsciousness
History of head injury
Inappropriate history

YELLOW

Recent mild pain
Recent injury

GREEN

BLUE

1	2	3	4	5

Notes accompanying apparently drunk

See also	Chart notes
Behaving strangely Collapse Head injury	This is a presentation defined flow diagram. A large number of patients attend for emergency treatment in an apparently drunken state. This chart implicitly recognises that not all these patients are drunk and is designed to ensure accurate identification and prioritisation of patients who are suffering from conditions which make them appear drunk, or from such severe drunkenness that their life is threatened. A number of general discriminators have been used including *Life threat*, *Conscious level in children* and *Blood glucose level.* Specific discriminators have been included to ensure that patients with an inadequate history of alcohol ingestion are seen rapidly and treated. If there is any doubt then the patient should be seen very urgently

Specific discriminators	Explanation
Hypoglycaemia	Glucose less than 3 mmol/l
Extreme aggression or agitation requiring immediate restraint	Aggression and agitation of such a degree that immediate restraint is required to manage the risk of harm to self or others
Altered conscious level *not* wholly attributable to alcohol	A patient who is not fully alert, with a history of alcohol ingestion, and in whom there may be other causes of reduced conscious level fulfils this discriminator definition
New neurological deficit less than 24 hrs old	Any loss of neurological function that has come on within the previous 24 hours. This might include altered or lost sensation, weakness of the limbs (either transiently or permanently) and alterations in bladder or bowel function
Inadequate history	If there is no clear and unequivocal history of acute alcohol ingestion, and if head injury, drug ingestion, underlying medical condition, etc. cannot be definitely excluded then the history is inadequate
Altered conscious level wholly attributable to alcohol	A patient who is not fully alert, with a clear history of alcohol ingestion and in whom there is no doubt that all other causes of reduced conscious level have been excluded fulfils this discriminator definition
New neurological deficit more than 24 hrs old	Any loss of neurological function including altered or lost sensation, weakness of the limbs (either transiently or permanently) and alterations in bladder or bowel function
History of unconsciousness	There may be a reliable witness who can state whether the patient was unconscious (and for how long). If not, a patient who is unable to remember the incident should be assumed to have been unconscious
History of head injury	A history of a recent physically traumatic event involving the head. Usually this will be reported by the patient but if the patient has been unconscious this history should be sought from a reliable witness
Recent injury	Any injury occurring within the last week

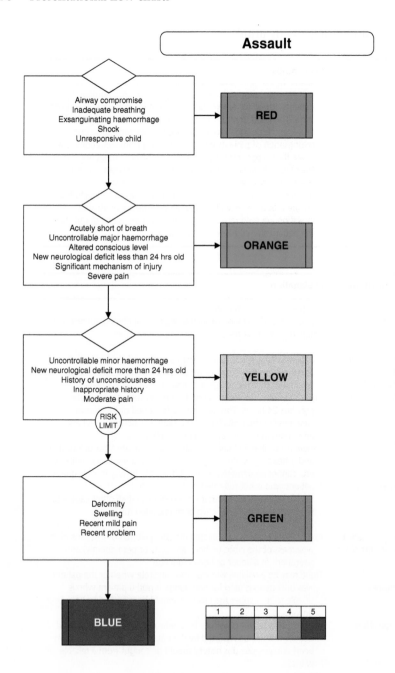

Assault

Airway compromise
Inadequate breathing
Exsanguinating haemorrhage
Shock
Unresponsive child

RED

Acutely short of breath
Uncontrollable major haemorrhage
Altered conscious level
New neurological deficit less than 24 hrs old
Significant mechanism of injury
Severe pain

ORANGE

Uncontrollable minor haemorrhage
New neurological deficit more than 24 hrs old
History of unconsciousness
Inappropriate history
Moderate pain

RISK LIMIT

YELLOW

Deformity
Swelling
Recent mild pain
Recent problem

GREEN

BLUE

Notes accompanying assault

See also	Chart notes
Head injury Torso injury Wounds	This is a presentation defined flow diagram. Assault is a common presentation, and patients with non-specific conditions following assault may be triaged using this chart. Patients who have specific injuries are better triaged using the charts that pertain to those injuries. A number of general discriminators are used including *Life threat*, *Haemorrhage* and *Pain*. Specific discriminators are included to identify patients who have a significant history of injury which may indicate a more urgent requirement for treatment

Specific discriminators	Explanation
Acutely short of breath	Shortness of breath that comes on suddenly, or a sudden exacerbation of chronic shortness of breath
New neurological deficit less than 24 hrs old	Any loss of neurological function that has come on within the previous 24 hours. This might include altered or lost sensation, weakness of the limbs (either transiently or permanently) and alterations in bladder or bowel function
Significant mechanism of injury	Penetrating injuries (stab or gunshot) and injuries with high energy transfer
New neurological deficit more than 24 hrs old	Any loss of neurological function including altered or lost sensation, weakness of the limbs (either transiently or permanently) and alterations in bladder or bowel function
History of unconsciousness	There may be a reliable witness who can state whether the patient was unconscious (and for how long). If not, a patient who is unable to remember the incident should be assumed to have been unconscious
Inappropriate history	When the history (story) given does not explain the physical findings it is termed inappropriate. This is important as it is a marker of safeguarding concerns in both adults and children
Deformity	This will always be subjective. Abnormal angulation or rotation is implied
Swelling	An abnormal increase in size

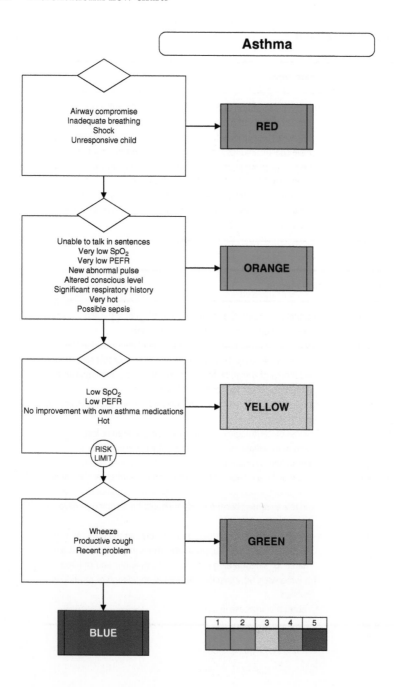

Notes accompanying asthma

See also	Chart notes

Allergy
Shortness of breath
  in adults
Shortness of breath
  in children
	This is a presentation defined flow diagram which is intended for use in patients who present with the symptoms and signs of known asthma. The severity of asthmatic patients at presentation varies from those whose lives are threatened to those requiring a repeat prescription of inhalers. A number of general discriminators are used including *Life threat, Conscious level (in adults and children)* and *Oxygen saturation.* Specific discriminators are included to indicate those signs and symptoms that indicate severe and life-threatening asthma

Specific discriminators	Explanation
Unable to talk in sentences	Patients who are so breathless that they cannot complete relatively short sentences in one breath
Very low SpO$_2$	This is a saturation of less than 95% on O$_2$ therapy or less than 92% on air
Very low PEFR	The PEFR predicted after consideration of the age and sex of the patient. Some patients may know their 'best' PEFR and this may be used. If the ratio of measured to predicted is less than 33% then this criterion is fulfilled
New abnormal pulse	A bradycardia (less than 60/min in adults), a tachycardia (more than 100/min in adults) or an irregular rhythm. Age-appropriate definitions of bradycardia and tachycardia should be used in children
Significant respiratory history	A history of previous life-threatening episodes of a respiratory condition (e.g. chronic obstructive pulmonary disease, COPD) is significant as is brittle asthma
Possible sepsis	Suspected sepsis in patients who present with altered mental state, low blood pressure (systolic less than 100) or raised respiratory rate (rate more than 22). In children, age specific physiological tools should be used to determine if possibly septic
Low SpO$_2$	This is a saturation of less than 95% on air
Low PEFR	The PEFR predicted after consideration of the age and sex of the patient. Some patients may know their 'best' PEFR and this may be used. If the ratio of measured to predicted is less than 50% then this criterion is fulfilled
No improvement with own asthma medications	This history should be available from the patient. A failure to improve with bronchodilator therapy given by the GP or paramedic is equally significant
Wheeze	This can be audible wheeze or a feeling of wheeze. Very severe airway obstruction is silent (no air can move)
Productive cough	A cough that is productive of phlegm, whatever the colour

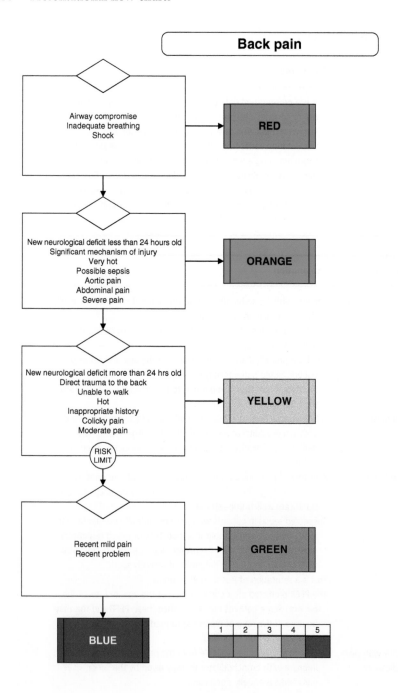

Notes accompanying back pain

See also	Chart notes
Abdominal pain in adults Abdominal pain in children Neck pain	This is a presentation defined flow diagram. Back pain may present to the Emergency Department either as an acute event or as an acute exacerbation of a chronic problem. A number of general discriminators are used including *Life threat*, *Pain* and *Temperature*. Specific discriminators have been selected in order to allow for appropriate categorisation of more urgent problems. In particular, discriminators are included to allow appropriate classification of abdominal aneurysm and patients with neurological signs and symptoms following disc prolapse

Specific discriminators	Explanation
New neurological deficit less than 24 hrs old	Any loss of neurological function that has come on within the previous 24 hours. This might include altered or lost sensation, weakness of the limbs (either transiently or permanently) and alterations in bladder or bowel function
Significant mechanism of injury	Penetrating injuries (stab or gunshot) and injuries with high energy transfer
Possible sepsis	Suspected sepsis in patients who present with altered mental state, low blood pressure (systolic less than 100) or raised respiratory rate (rate more than 22). In children, age specific physiological tools should be used to determine if possibly septic
Aortic pain	The onset of symptoms is sudden and the leading symptom is severe abdominal or chest pain. The pain may be described as sharp, stabbing or ripping in character. Classically aortic chest pain is felt around the sternum and then radiates to the shoulder blades, aortic abdominal pain is felt in the centre of the abdomen and radiates to the back. The pain may get better or even vanish and then recur elsewhere. Over time, pain may also be felt in the arms, neck, lower jaw, stomach or hips
Abdominal pain	Any pain felt in the abdomen. Abdominal pain associated with back pain may indicate abdominal aortic aneurysm, while association with PV bleeding may indicate ectopic pregnancy or miscarriage
New neurological deficit more than 24 hrs old	Any loss of neurological function including altered or lost sensation, weakness of the limbs (either transiently or permanently) and alterations in bladder or bowel function
Direct trauma to the back	This may be top to bottom (loading), for instance when people fall and land on their feet, bending (forwards, backwards or to the side) or twisting
Unable to walk	It is important to try and distinguish between patients who have pain and difficulty walking and those who *cannot* walk. Only the latter can be said to be unable to walk
Inappropriate history	When the history (story) given does not explain the physical findings it is termed inappropriate. This is important as it is a marker of safeguarding concerns in both adults and children
Colicky pain	Pain that comes and goes in waves. Renal colic tends to come and go over 20 minutes or so

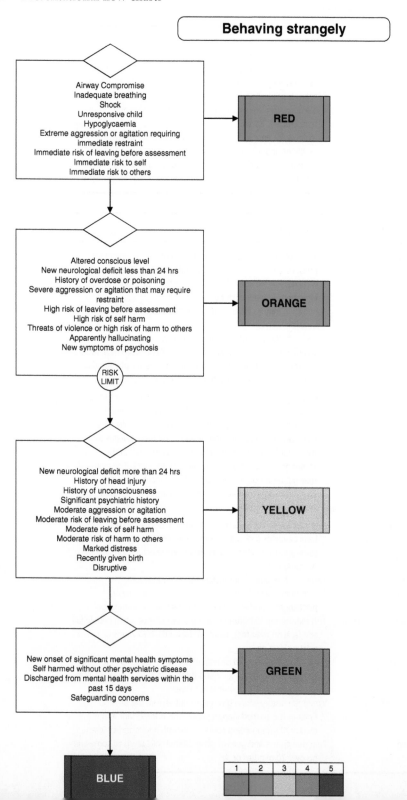

Behaving strangely

Airway Compromise
Inadequate breathing
Shock
Unresponsive child
Hypoglycaemia
Extreme aggression or agitation requiring
immediate restraint
Immediate risk of leaving before assessment
Immediate risk to self
Immediate risk to others

RED

Altered conscious level
New neurological deficit less than 24 hrs
History of overdose or poisoning
Severe aggression or agitation that may require
restraint
High risk of leaving before assessment
High risk of self harm
Threats of violence or high risk of harm to others
Apparently hallucinating
New symptoms of psychosis

ORANGE

RISK
LIMIT

New neurological deficit more than 24 hrs
History of head injury
History of unconsciousness
Significant psychiatric history
Moderate aggression or agitation
Moderate risk of leaving before assessment
Moderate risk of self harm
Moderate risk of harm to others
Marked distress
Recently given birth
Disruptive

YELLOW

New onset of significant mental health symptoms
Self harmed without other psychiatric disease
Discharged from mental health services within the
past 15 days
Safeguarding concerns

GREEN

BLUE

| 1 | 2 | 3 | 4 | 5 |

Notes accompanying behaving strangely

See also	Chart notes
Apparently drunk Mental illness	This is a presentation defined flow diagram. Patients who are behaving strangely may have either a psychiatric or a physical cause for their presentation. This chart is designed to allow the accurate prioritisation of both these groups of patients. A number of general discriminators have been used including *Life threat* and *Conscious level.* Specific discriminators are used and in particular the concepts of risk of harm to others and risks of self-harm are introduced

Specific discriminators	Explanation
Hypoglycaemia	Glucose less than 3 mmol/l
New neurological deficit less than 24 hrs old	Any loss of neurological function that has come on within the previous 24 hours. This might include altered or lost sensation, weakness of the limbs (either transiently or permanently) and alterations in bladder or bowel function
History of overdose or poisoning	This information may come from others or may be deduced if medication is missing
High risk of self harm	An initial view of the risk of harm to self can be formed by considering the patient's behaviour. Patients who are threatening to harm themselves and who are actively seeking the means to do so are at high risk
Threats of violence or high risk of harm to others	An initial view of the risk of harm to others can be judged by looking at posture (tense, clenched), speech (loud, using threatening words) and motor behaviour (restless, pacing, lunging at others). High risk should be assumed if potential victims are available and inadequate controls are in place
History of head injury	A history of a recent physically traumatic event involving the head. Usually this will be reported by the patient but if the patient has been unconscious this history should be sought from a reliable witness
History of unconsciousness	There may be a reliable witness who can state whether the patient was unconscious (and for how long). If not, a patient who is unable to remember the incident should be assumed to have been unconscious
Significant psychiatric history	A history of a major psychiatric illness or event
Moderate risk of self harm	An initial view of the risk of harm to self can be formed by considering the patient's behaviour. Patients without a significant history of self harm, who are not actively trying to harm themselves, but who profess the desire to harm themselves are at moderate risk
Moderate risk of harm to others	An initial view of the risk of harm to others can be judged by looking at posture (tense, clenched), speech (loud, using threatening words) and motor behaviour (restless, pacing, lunging at others). Moderate risk should be assumed if there is any indication of potential harm to others
Recently given birth	A woman who has given birth within the past 3 months
Discharged from mental health services within the past 15 days	Any patient who has been discharged from an active period of care under mental health services (in hospital or in the community) within the past 15 days

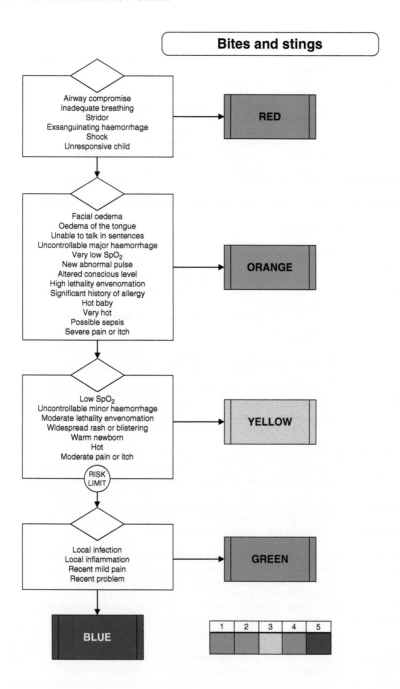

Bites and stings

Airway compromise
Inadequate breathing
Stridor
Exsanguinating haemorrhage
Shock
Unresponsive child

RED

Facial oedema
Oedema of the tongue
Unable to talk in sentences
Uncontrollable major haemorrhage
Very low SpO_2
New abnormal pulse
Altered conscious level
High lethality envenomation
Significant history of allergy
Hot baby
Very hot
Possible sepsis
Severe pain or itch

ORANGE

Low SpO_2
Uncontrollable minor haemorrhage
Moderate lethality envenomation
Widespread rash or blistering
Warm newborn
Hot
Moderate pain or itch

RISK
LIMIT

YELLOW

Local infection
Local inflammation
Recent mild pain
Recent problem

GREEN

BLUE

1	2	3	4	5

Notes accompanying bites and stings

See also	Chart notes
Abscesses and local infections Allergy	This is a presentation defined flow diagram designed to allow accurate prioritisation of patients who present following bites and stings. Bites may, of course, range from those delivered by insects to those delivered by large animals; therefore, there is a complete range of priority covered by this presentation. A number of general discriminators are used including *Life threat*, *Haemorrhage* and *Pain*. Specific discriminators have been added to the chart to allow accurate identification of patients requiring more urgent treatment because of more severe injury or the development of allergic reactions

Specific discriminators	Explanation
Stridor	This may be an inspiratory or expiratory noise, or both. Stridor is heard best on breathing with the mouth open
Facial oedema	Diffuse swelling around the face, usually involving the lips
Oedema of the tongue	Swelling of the tongue of any degree
Unable to talk in sentences	Patients who are so breathless that they cannot complete relatively short sentences in one breath
Very low SpO_2	This is a saturation of less than 95% on O_2 therapy or less than 92% on air
High lethality envenomation	Lethality is the potential of the envenomation to cause harm. Local knowledge may allow identification of the venomous creature, but advice may be required. If in doubt, assume a high risk
Significant history of allergy	A known sensitivity with severe reaction (e.g. to nuts or bee sting) is significant
Possible sepsis	Suspected sepsis in patients who present with altered mental state, low blood pressure (systolic less than 100) or raised respiratory rate (rate more than 22). In children, age specific physiological tools should be used to determine if possibly septic
Low SpO_2	This is a saturation of less than 95% on air
Moderate lethality envenomation	Lethality is the potential of the substance taken to cause serious illness or death. Advice from a poisons centre may be required to establish the level of risk to the patient
Widespread rash or blistering	Any discharging or blistering eruption covering more than 10% of the body surface area
Local infection	Local infection usually manifests as inflammation (pain, swelling and redness) confined to a particular site or area, with or without a collection of pus
Local inflammation	Local inflammation will involve pain, swelling and redness confined to a particular site or area

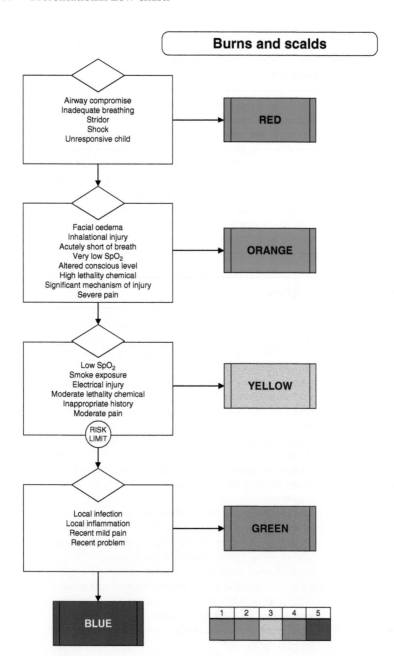

Burns and scalds

Airway compromise
Inadequate breathing
Stridor
Shock
Unresponsive child

RED

Facial oedema
Inhalational injury
Acutely short of breath
Very low SpO$_2$
Altered conscious level
High lethality chemical
Significant mechanism of injury
Severe pain

ORANGE

Low SpO$_2$
Smoke exposure
Electrical injury
Moderate lethality chemical
Inappropriate history
Moderate pain

RISK
LIMIT

YELLOW

Local infection
Local inflammation
Recent mild pain
Recent problem

GREEN

BLUE

1	2	3	4	5

Notes accompanying burns and scalds

See also	Chart notes
	This is a presentation defined flow diagram. There is a complete range of severity with this presentation and the chart has been designed to allow accurate identification of patients within each category. A number of general discriminators are used including *Life threat*, *Conscious level* and *Pain*. Specific discriminators have been added to allow identification of patients who have suffered inhalation injury, and those in whom the mechanism suggests that further investigation and treatment may be appropriate

Specific discriminators	Explanation
Stridor	This may be an inspiratory or expiratory noise, or both. Stridor is heard best on breathing with the mouth open
Facial oedema	Diffuse swelling around the face, usually involving the lips
Inhalational injury	A history of being confined in a smoke-filled space is the most reliable indicator of smoke inhalation. Carbon deposits around the mouth and nose and hoarse voice may present. History is also the most reliable way of diagnosing inhalation of chemicals – there will not necessarily be any signs
Acutely short of breath	Shortness of breath that comes on suddenly, or a sudden exacerbation of chronic shortness of breath
Very low SpO_2	This is a saturation of less than 95% on O_2 therapy or less than 92% on air
High lethality chemical	Lethality is the potential of the chemical to cause harm. Advice may be required to establish the level of risk. If in doubt, assume a high risk
Significant mechanism of injury	Penetrating injuries (stab or gunshot) and injuries with high energy transfer
Low SpO_2	This is a saturation of less than 95% on air
Smoke exposure	Smoke inhalation should be assumed if the patient has been confined in a smoke-filled space. Physical signs such as oral or nasal soot are less reliable but significant if present
Electrical injury	Any injury caused or possibly caused by an electric current. This includes AC and DC and both artificial and natural sources
Moderate lethality chemical	Lethality is the potential of the chemical to cause harm. Advice may be required to establish the level of risk. If in doubt, assume a high risk
Inappropriate history	When the history (story) given does not explain the physical findings it is termed inappropriate. This is important as it is a marker of safeguarding concerns in both adults and children
Local infection	Local infection usually manifests as inflammation (pain, swelling and redness) confined to a particular site or area, with or without a collection of pus
Local inflammation	Local inflammation will involve pain, swelling and redness confined to a particular site or area

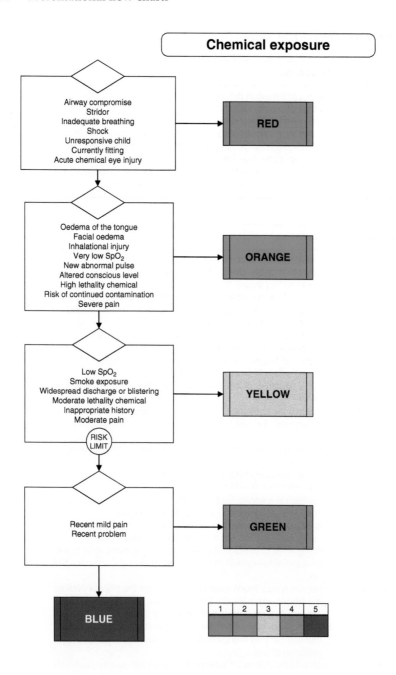

Chemical exposure

Airway compromise
Stridor
Inadequate breathing
Shock
Unresponsive child
Currently fitting
Acute chemical eye injury

RED

Oedema of the tongue
Facial oedema
Inhalational injury
Very low SpO$_2$
New abnormal pulse
Altered conscious level
High lethality chemical
Risk of continued contamination
Severe pain

ORANGE

Low SpO$_2$
Smoke exposure
Widespread discharge or blistering
Moderate lethality chemical
Inappropriate history
Moderate pain

YELLOW

RISK
LIMIT

Recent mild pain
Recent problem

GREEN

BLUE

Notes accompanying chemical exposure

See also	Chart notes

Overdose and poisoning
Shortness of breath
  in adults
Shortness of breath
  in children
	This is a presentation defined flow diagram. While this presentation is not common it is important because it is often the chief complaint of the patient. The signs and symptoms do not necessarily fit easily into any other presentational group. A number of general discriminators are used including *Life threat*, *Conscious level*, *Pain* and *Oxygen saturation*. Specific discriminators, which include those for the shortness of breath, have been added to appropriate categories. *Acute chemical eye injury* appears in the RED category and *Risk of continued contamination* appears in the ORANGE

Specific discriminators	Explanation
Stridor	This may be an inspiratory or expiratory noise, or both. Stridor is heard best on breathing with the mouth open
Acute chemical eye injury	Any substance splashed into or placed into the eye within the past 12 hours that caused stinging, burning or reduced vision should be assumed to be have caused chemical injury
Oedema of the tongue	Swelling of the tongue of any degree
Facial oedema	Diffuse swelling around the face, usually involving the lips
Inhalational injury	A history of being confined in a smoke-filled space is the most reliable indicator of smoke inhalation. Carbon deposits around the mouth and nose and hoarse voice may be present. History is also the most reliable way of diagnosing inhalation of chemicals – there will not necessarily be any signs
Very low SpO$_2$	This is a saturation of less than 95% on O$_2$ therapy or less than 92% on air
New abnormal pulse	A bradycardia (less than 60/min in adults), a tachycardia (more than 100/min in adults) or an irregular rhythm. Age-appropriate definitions of bradycardia and tachycardia should be used in children
High lethality chemical	Lethality is the potential of the chemical to cause harm. Advice may be required to establish the level of risk. If in doubt, assume a high risk
Risk of continued contamination	If chemical exposure is likely to continue (usually due to lack of adequate decontamination) then this discriminator applies. Risks to health care workers must not be forgotten if this situation occurs
Low SpO$_2$	This is a saturation of less than 95% on air
Smoke exposure	Smoke inhalation should be assumed if the patient has been confined in a smoke-filled space. Physical signs such as oral or nasal soot are less reliable but significant if present
Widespread discharge or blistering	Any discharging or blistering eruption covering more than 10% of the body surface area
Moderate lethality chemical	Lethality is the potential of the chemical to cause harm. Advice may be required to establish the level of risk. If in doubt, assume a high risk
Inappropriate history	When the history (story) given does not explain the physical findings it is termed inappropriate. This is important as it is a marker of safeguarding concerns in both adults and children

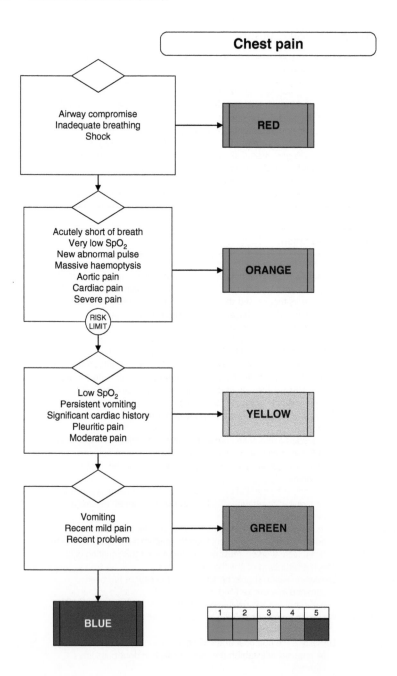

Notes accompanying chest pain

See also	Chart notes
	This is a presentation defined flow diagram. Chest pain is a common presentation to Emergency Departments, forming some 2–5% of all patient contacts. Causes of chest pain may vary from acute myocardial infraction to muscular irritation, and appropriate categorisation is paramount. A number of general discriminators are used including *Life threat* and *Pain*. Specific discriminators include the nature and severity of pain (cardiac or pleuritic) and abnormalities of pulse

Specific discriminators	Explanation
Acutely short of breath	Shortness of breath that comes on suddenly, or a sudden exacerbation of chronic shortness of breath
Very low SpO$_2$	This is a saturation of less than 95% on O$_2$ therapy or less than 92% on air
New abnormal pulse	A bradycardia (less than 60/min in adults), a tachycardia (more than 100/min in adults) or an irregular rhythm. Age-appropriate definitions of bradycardia and tachycardia should be used in children
Massive haemoptysis	Coughing up large amounts of fresh or clotted blood. Not to be confused with streaks of blood in saliva
Aortic Pain	The onset of symptoms is sudded and the leading symptom is severe abdominal or chest pain. The pain may be described as sharp, stabbing or ripping in character. Classically aortic chest pain is felt around the sternum and then radiates to the shoulder blades, aortic abdominal pain is felt in the centre of the abdomen and radiates to the back. The pain may get better or even vanish and then recur elsewhere. Over time, pain may also be felt in the arms, neck, lower jaw, stomach or hips
Cardiac pain	Classically a severe dull 'gripping' or 'heavy' pain in the centre of the chest, radiating to the left arm or to the neck. May be associated with sweating and nausea
Low SpO$_2$	This is a saturation of less than 95% on air
Persistent vomiting	Vomiting that is continuous or that occurs without any respite between episodes
Significant cardiac history	A known recurrent dysrhythmia that has life-threatening effects is significant, as is a known cardiac condition which may deteriorate rapidly
Pleuritic pain	A sharp, localised pain in the chest that worsens on breathing, coughing or sneezing
Vomiting	Any emesis

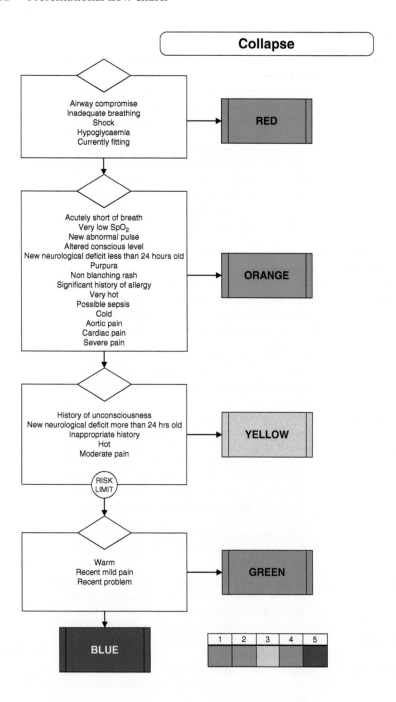

Notes accompanying collapse

See also	Chart notes
Apparently drunk Falls Fits Unwell adult	This is a presentation defined flow diagram. Presentation with collapse is not uncommon in an Emergency Department and this chart is designed to allow rapid triage of patients who present in this way. A number of general discriminators are used including *Life threat*, *Conscious level*, *Pain* and *Temperature*. Specific discriminators have been added to the chart to try and rule out more serious pathology. As with all charts, those pathologies (such as myocardial infarction) which can potentially benefit from early intervention are deliberately categorised highly

Specific discriminators	Explanation
Hypoglycaemia	Glucose less than 3 mmol/l
Acutely short of breath	Shortness of breath that comes on suddenly, or a sudden exacerbation of chronic shortness of breath
New abnormal pulse	A bradycardia (less than 60/min in adults), a tachycardia (more than 100/min in adults) or an irregular rhythm. Age-appropriate definitions of bradycardia and tachycardia should be used in children
New neurological deficit less than 24 hrs old	Any loss of neurological function that has come on within the previous 24 hours. This might include altered or lost sensation, weakness of the limbs (either transiently or permanently) and alterations in bladder or bowel function
Purpura	A rash on any part of the body that is caused by small haemorrhages under the skin. A purpuric rash does not blanch (go white) when pressure is applied to it
Non-blanching rash	A rash that does not blanch (go white) when pressure is applied to it. Often tested using a glass tumbler to apply pressure as any colour change can be observed through the bottom of the tumbler
Significant history of allergy	A known sensitivity with severe reaction (e.g. to nuts or bee sting) is significant
Possible sepsis	Suspected sepsis in patients who present with altered mental state, low blood pressure (systolic less than 100) or raised respiratory rate (rate more than 22). In children, age specific physiological tools should be used to determine if possibly septic
Aortic Pain	The onset of symptoms is sudded and the leading symptom is severe abdominal or chest pain. The pain may be described as sharp, stabbing or ripping in character. Classically aortic chest pain is felt around the sternum and then radiates to the shoulder blades, aortic abdominal pain is felt in the centre of the abdomen and radiates to the back. The pain may get better or even vanish and then recur elsewhere. Over time, pain may also be felt in the arms, neck, lower jaw, stomach or hips
Cardiac pain	Classically a severe dull 'gripping' or 'heavy' pain in the centre of the chest, radiating to the left arm or to the neck. May be associated with sweating and nausea
New neurological deficit more than 24 hrs old	Any loss of neurological function including altered or lost sensation, weakness of the limbs (either transiently or permanently) and alterations in bladder or bowel function
Inappropriate history	When the history (story) given does not explain the physical findings it is termed inappropriate. This is important as it is a marker of safeguarding concerns in both adults and children

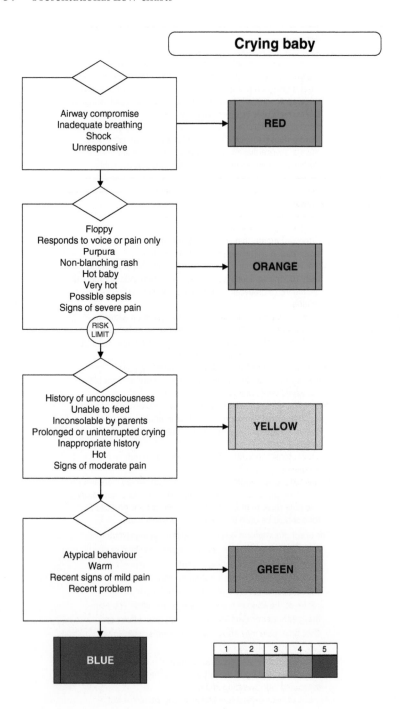

Crying baby

Airway compromise
Inadequate breathing
Shock
Unresponsive

RED

Floppy
Responds to voice or pain only
Purpura
Non-blanching rash
Hot baby
Very hot
Possible sepsis
Signs of severe pain

ORANGE

RISK LIMIT

History of unconsciousness
Unable to feed
Inconsolable by parents
Prolonged or uninterrupted crying
Inappropriate history
Hot
Signs of moderate pain

YELLOW

Atypical behaviour
Warm
Recent signs of mild pain
Recent problem

GREEN

BLUE

| 1 | 2 | 3 | 4 | 5 |

Notes accompanying crying baby

See also	Chart notes
Unwell baby Unwell child Unwell newborn Worried parent	This is a presentation defined flow diagram. This chart has been designed to allow accurate prioritisation of children who are presented by their parents with a chief complaint of crying. A number of general discriminators have been used including *Life threat, Conscious level* and *Pain*. Specific discriminators include those that allow recognition of more specific pathologies such as septicaemia, or that indicate that a more serious pathology might exist The risk limit sits between ORANGE and YELLOW and therefore no children can be categorised as YELLOW, GREEN or BLUE until all the specific and general discriminators outlined under the RED and ORANGE categories have been specifically excluded. This may take longer than the time available for initial assessment. If the patient is under 28 days, the Unwell Newborn chart should be used

Specific discriminators	Explanation
Floppy	Parents may describe their children as floppy. Tone is generally reduced – the most noticeable sign is often lolling of the head
Responds to pain	Response to a painful stimulus. Standard peripheral stimuli should be used – a pencil or pen is used to apply pressure to the finger nail bed. This stimulus should not be applied to the toes since a spinal reflex may cause flexion even in brain death. Supraorbital ridge pressure should not be used since reflex grimacing may occur
Responds to voice	Response to a vocal stimulus. It is not necessary to shout the patient's name. Children may fail to respond because they are afraid
Purpura	A rash on any part of the body that is caused by small haemorrhages under the skin. A purpuric rash does not blanch (go white) when pressure is applied to it
Non-blanching rash	A rash that does not blanch (go white) when pressure is applied to it. Often tested using a glass tumbler to apply pressure as any colour change can be observed through the bottom of the tumbler
Possible sepsis	Suspected sepsis in patients who present with altered mental state, low blood pressure (systolic less than 100) or raised respiratory rate (rate more than 22). In children, age specific physiological tools should be used to determine if possibly septic
Signs of severe pain	Young children and babies in severe pain cannot complain. They will usually cry out continuously and inconsolably and be tachycardic. They may well exhibit signs such as pallor and sweating
Unable to feed	This is usually reported by the parents. Children who will not take any solid or liquid (as appropriate) by mouth
Inconsolable by parents	Children whose crying or distress does not respond to attempts by their parents to comfort them
Prolonged or uninterrupted crying	A child who has cried continuously for 2 hours or more
Inappropriate history	When the history (story) given does not explain the physical findings it is termed inappropriate. This is important as it is a marker of safeguarding concerns in both adults and children
Signs of moderate pain	Young children and babies in moderate pain cannot complain. They will usually cry intermittently and are often intermittently consolable
Atypical behaviour	A child who is behaving in a way that is not usual in the given situation. The carers will often volunteer this information. Such children are often referred to as fractious or 'out of sorts'

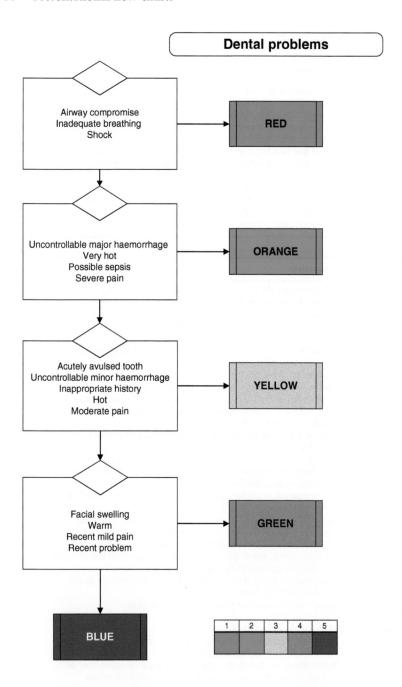

Dental problems

Notes accompanying dental problems

See also	Chart notes
Facial problems	This is a presentation defined flow diagram designed to allow accurate prioritisation of patients presenting problems affecting the teeth or gums. A number of general discriminators have been used including *Life threat, Pain, Haemorrhage* and *Temperature*. Acute avulsion of a tooth has been included in the urgent (YELLOW) category since speed of reimplantation affects outcome. It is important to ensure that preconceptions about disposal do not affect accurate triage of patients with these presentations

Specific discriminators	Explanation
Possible sepsis	Suspected sepsis in patients who present with altered mental state, low blood pressure (systolic less than 100) or raised respiratory rate (rate more than 22). In children, age specific physiological tools should be used to determine if possibly septic
Acutely avulsed tooth	A tooth that has been avulsed intact within the previous 24 hours
Inappropriate history	When the history (story) given does not explain the physical findings it is termed inappropriate. This is important as it is a marker of safeguarding concerns in both adults and children
Facial swelling	Swelling around the face which may be localised or diffuse

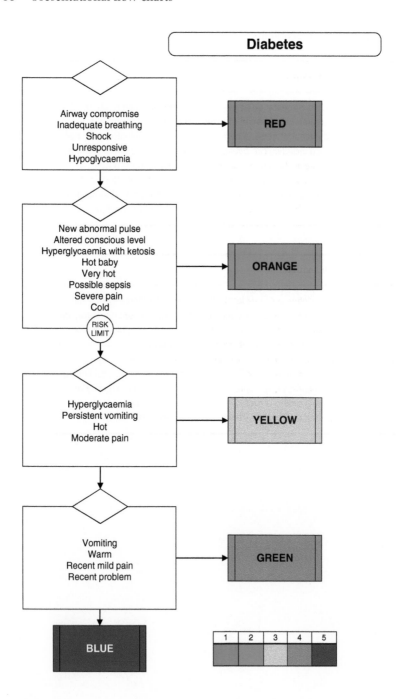

Diabetes

Airway compromise
Inadequate breathing
Shock
Unresponsive
Hypoglycaemia

RED

New abnormal pulse
Altered conscious level
Hyperglycaemia with ketosis
Hot baby
Very hot
Possible sepsis
Severe pain
Cold

ORANGE

RISK LIMIT

Hyperglycaemia
Persistent vomiting
Hot
Moderate pain

YELLOW

Vomiting
Warm
Recent mild pain
Recent problem

GREEN

BLUE

| 1 | 2 | 3 | 4 | 5 |

Notes accompanying diabetes

See also	Chart notes
Unwell newborn	This is a presentation defined flow diagram designed to allow categorisation of patients who present with known cases of diabetes. A number of general discriminators are used including *Life threat*, *Conscious level (both adult and child)*, *Blood glucose level* and *Temperature*. If the patient is under 28 days, the Unwell Newborn chart should be used

Specific discriminators	Explanation
Hypoglycaemia	Glucose less than 3 mmol/l
Hyperglycaemia with ketosis	Glucose greater than 11 mmol/l with urinary ketones or signs of acidosis (deep sighing respiration, etc.)
Possible sepsis	Suspected sepsis in patients who present with altered mental state, low blood pressure (systolic less than 100) or raised respiratory rate (rate more than 22). In children, age specific physiological tools should be used to determine if possibly septic
Hyperglycaemia	Glucose greater than 17 mmol/l
Persistent vomiting	Vomiting that is continuous or that occurs without any respite between episodes
Vomiting	Any emesis

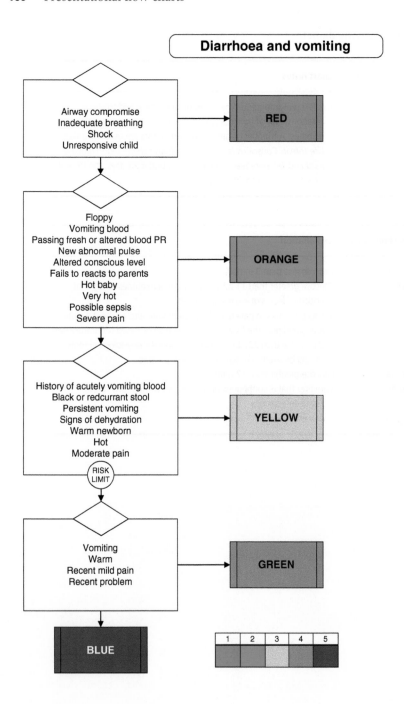

Diarrhoea and vomiting

Airway compromise
Inadequate breathing
Shock
Unresponsive child

RED

Floppy
Vomiting blood
Passing fresh or altered blood PR
New abnormal pulse
Altered conscious level
Fails to reacts to parents
Hot baby
Very hot
Possible sepsis
Severe pain

ORANGE

History of acutely vomiting blood
Black or redcurrant stool
Persistent vomiting
Signs of dehydration
Warm newborn
Hot
Moderate pain

RISK LIMIT

YELLOW

Vomiting
Warm
Recent mild pain
Recent problem

GREEN

BLUE

| 1 | 2 | 3 | 4 | 5 |

Notes accompanying diarrhoea and vomiting

See also	Chart notes
Abdominal pain in adults Abdominal pain in children GI bleeding	This is a presentation defined flow diagram designed to allow categorisation of patients who present with diarrhoea and/or vomiting. Most patients who present with diarrhoea or vomiting do not have high priority. However, a number may have serious underlying pathology. A number of general discriminators are used including *Life threat* and *Pain*. Specific discriminators have been included to ensure that patients suffering from GI bleeding, and those with dehydration and other severe effects of diarrhoea and vomiting, are included in the appropriate categories

Specific discriminators	Explanation
Floppy	Parents may describe their children as floppy. Tone is generally reduced – the most noticeable sign is often lolling of the head
Fails to react to parents	Failure to react in any way to a parent's face or voice. Abnormal reactions and apparent lack of recognition of a parent are also worrying signs
Vomiting blood	Vomited blood may be fresh (bright or dark red) or coffee ground in appearance
Passing fresh or altered blood PR	In active massive GI bleeding dark red blood will be passed PR. As GI transit time increases this becomes darker, eventually becoming melaena
Possible sepsis	Suspected sepsis in patients who present with altered mental state, low blood pressure (systolic less than 100) or raised respiratory rate (rate more than 22). In children, age specific physiological tools should be used to determine if possibly septic
History of acutely vomiting blood	Frank haematemesis, vomiting of altered blood (coffee ground) or of blood mixed in the vomit within the past 24 hours
Black or redcurrant stool	Any blackness fulfils the criteria of black stool while a dark red stool, classically seen in intussusceptions, is redcurrant stool
Persistent vomiting	Vomiting that is continuous or that occurs without any respite between episodes
Signs of dehydration	These include dry tongue, sunken eyes, decreased skin turgor and, in small babies, a sunken anterior fontanelle. Usually associated with a low urine output
Vomiting	Any emesis

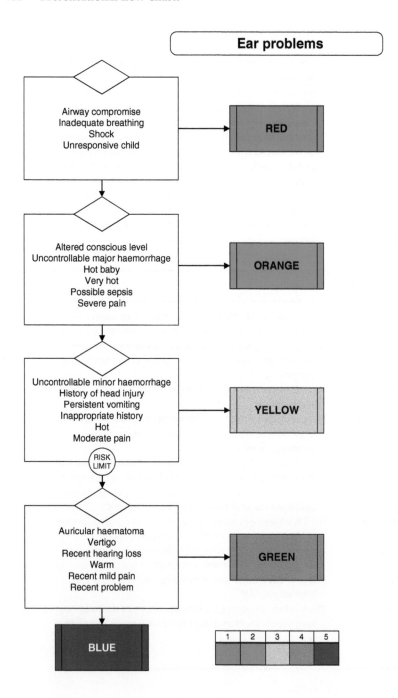

Ear problems

Airway compromise
Inadequate breathing
Shock
Unresponsive child
→ RED

Altered conscious level
Uncontrollable major haemorrhage
Hot baby
Very hot
Possible sepsis
Severe pain
→ ORANGE

Uncontrollable minor haemorrhage
History of head injury
Persistent vomiting
Inappropriate history
Hot
Moderate pain
→ YELLOW

RISK LIMIT

Auricular haematoma
Vertigo
Recent hearing loss
Warm
Recent mild pain
Recent problem
→ GREEN

BLUE

1	2	3	4	5

Notes accompanying ear problems

See also	Chart notes
Facial problems Head injury Unwell newborn	This is a presentation defined flow diagram designed to allow accurate prioritisation of patients presenting with conditions affecting the ear. A number of general discriminators are used including *Life threat*, *Pain*, *Haemorrhage* and *Temperature*. If the patient is under 28 days, the Unwell Newborn chart should be used

Specific discriminators	Explanation
Possible sepsis	Suspected sepsis in patients who present with altered mental state, low blood pressure (systolic less than 100) or raised respiratory rate (rate more than 22). In children, age specific physiological tools should be used to determine if possibly septic
History of head injury	A history of a recent physically traumatic event involving the head. Usually this will be reported by the patient but if the patient has been unconscious this history should be sought from a reliable witness
Persistent vomiting	Vomiting that is continuous or that occurs without any respite between episodes
Inappropriate history	When the history (story) given does not explain the physical findings it is termed inappropriate. This is important as it is a marker of safeguarding concerns in both adults and children
Auricular haematoma	A tense haematoma (usually post traumatic) in the outer ear
Vertigo	An acute feeling of spinning or dizziness, possibly accompanied by nausea and vomiting
Recent hearing loss	Loss of hearing in one or both ears within the previous week

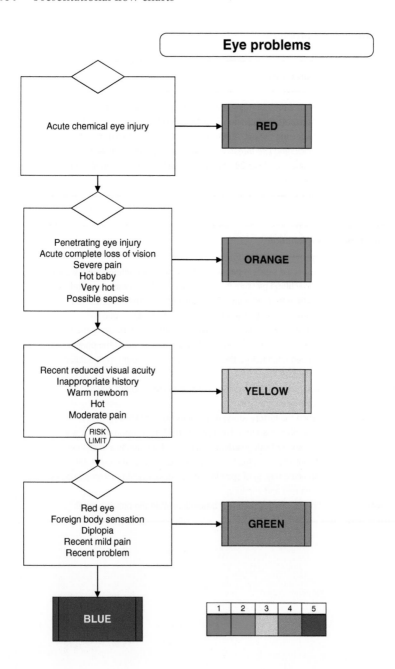

Eye problems

Acute chemical eye injury → **RED**

Penetrating eye injury
Acute complete loss of vision
Severe pain
Hot baby
Very hot
Possible sepsis
→ **ORANGE**

Recent reduced visual acuity
Inappropriate history
Warm newborn
Hot
Moderate pain
RISK LIMIT
→ **YELLOW**

Red eye
Foreign body sensation
Diplopia
Recent mild pain
Recent problem
→ **GREEN**

BLUE

1	2	3	4	5

Notes accompanying eye problems

See also	Chart notes
Facial problems	This is a presentation defined flow diagram designed to allow accurate prioritisation of patients attending with conditions affecting the eye. *Pain* is used as a general discriminator. A number of specific discriminators have been used including a history of *Acute chemical injury*, which indicates that immediate action is required, a history of *Penetrating eye injury* or sudden or *Acute complete loss of vision* and an assessment of visual acuity

Specific discriminators	Explanation
Acute chemical eye injury	Any substance splashed into or placed into the eye within the past 12 hours that caused stinging, burning or reduced vision should be assumed to have caused chemical injury
Penetrating eye injury	A recent physically traumatic event involving penetration of the globe
Acute complete loss of vision	Loss of vision in one or both eyes within the preceding 24 hours that has not returned to normal
Possible sepsis	Suspected sepsis in patients who present with altered mental state, low blood pressure (systolic less than 100) or raised respiratory rate (rate more than 22). In children, age specific physiological tools should be used to determine if possibly septic
Recent reduced visual acuity	Any reduction in corrected visual acuity within the past 7 days
Inappropriate history	When the history (story) given does not explain the physical findings it is termed inappropriate. This is important as it is a marker of safeguarding concerns in both adults and children
Red eye	Any redness to the eye. A red eye may be painful or painless and may be complete or partial
Foreign body sensation	A sensation of something in the eye, often expressed as scraping or grittiness
Diplopia	Double vision that resolves when one eye is closed

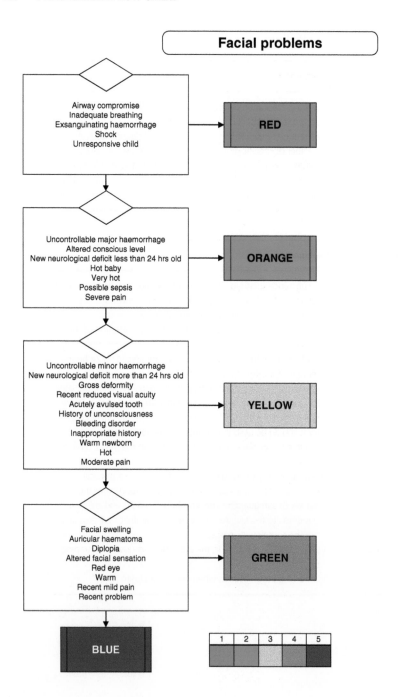

Facial problems

Airway compromise
Inadequate breathing
Exsanguinating haemorrhage
Shock
Unresponsive child

RED

Uncontrollable major haemorrhage
Altered conscious level
New neurological deficit less than 24 hrs old
Hot baby
Very hot
Possible sepsis
Severe pain

ORANGE

Uncontrollable minor haemorrhage
New neurological deficit more than 24 hrs old
Gross deformity
Recent reduced visual acuity
Acutely avulsed tooth
History of unconsciousness
Bleeding disorder
Inappropriate history
Warm newborn
Hot
Moderate pain

YELLOW

Facial swelling
Auricular haematoma
Diplopia
Altered facial sensation
Red eye
Warm
Recent mild pain
Recent problem

GREEN

BLUE

1	2	3	4	5

Notes accompanying facial problems

See also	Chart notes
Dental problems Ear problems Eye problems Head injury	This presentation defined flow diagram has been designed to allow accurate prioritisation of patients attending with problems affecting the face. A number of general discriminators have been used including *Life threat*, *Haemorrhage* and *Pain*

Specific discriminators	Explanation
New neurological deficit less than 24 hrs old	Any loss of neurological function that has come on within the previous 24 hours. This might include altered or lost sensation, weakness of the limbs (either transiently or permanently) and alterations in bladder or bowel function
Possible sepsis	Suspected sepsis in patients who present with altered mental state, low blood pressure (systolic less than 100) or raised respiratory rate (rate more than 22). In children, age specific physiological tools should be used to determine if possibly septic
New neurological deficit more than 24 hrs old	Any loss of neurological function including altered or lost sensation, weakness of the limbs (either transiently or permanently) and alterations in bladder or bowel function
Gross deformity	This will always be subjective. Gross and abnormal angulation or rotation is implied
Recent reduced visual acuity	Any reduction in corrected visual acuity within the past 7 days
Acutely avulsed tooth	A tooth that has been avulsed intact within the previous 24 hours
History of unconsciousness	There may be a reliable witness who can state whether the patient was unconscious (and for how long). If not, a patient who is unable to remember the incident should be assumed to have been unconscious
Bleeding disorder	Congenital or acquired bleeding disorder
Inappropriate history	When the history (story) given does not explain the physical findings it is termed inappropriate. This is important as it is a marker of safeguarding concerns in both adults and children
Facial swelling	Swelling around the face which may be localised or diffuse
Auricular haematoma	A tense haematoma (usually post traumatic) in the outer ear
Diplopia	Double vision that resolves when one eye is closed
Altered facial sensation	Any alteration of sensation on the face
Red eye	Any redness to the eye. A red eye may be painful or painless and may be complete or partial

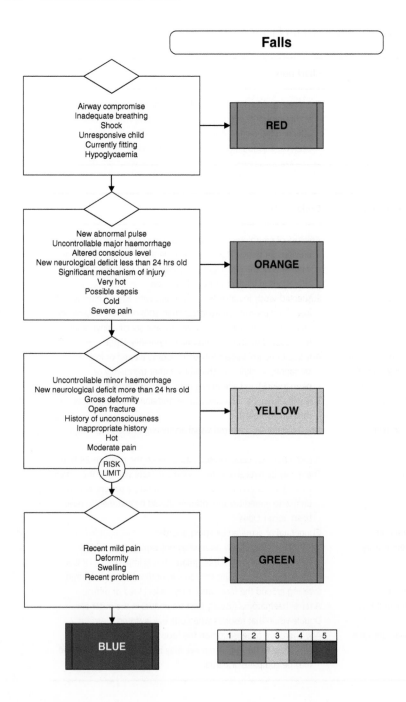

Falls

Airway compromise
Inadequate breathing
Shock
Unresponsive child
Currently fitting
Hypoglycaemia

RED

New abnormal pulse
Uncontrollable major haemorrhage
Altered conscious level
New neurological deficit less than 24 hrs old
Significant mechanism of injury
Very hot
Possible sepsis
Cold
Severe pain

ORANGE

Uncontrollable minor haemorrhage
New neurological deficit more than 24 hrs old
Gross deformity
Open fracture
History of unconsciousness
Inappropriate history
Hot
Moderate pain

RISK LIMIT

YELLOW

Recent mild pain
Deformity
Swelling
Recent problem

GREEN

BLUE

| 1 | 2 | 3 | 4 | 5 |

Notes accompanying falls

See also	Chart notes
Collapse	This is a presentation defined flow diagram. Many patients who present with a history of falls have suffered trauma as a result, and their priority will reflect the injuries suffered. Some, however, may have had a serious underlying pathology that caused them to fall, or may have developed complications after falling. This chart is designed to allow accurate prioritisation whether the injury or underlying cause is more pressing. A number of general discriminators have been included to ensure that patients suffering from serious underlying conditions or limb-threatening injuries are given a high priority

Specific discriminators	Explanation
Hypoglycaemia	Glucose less than 3 mmol/l
New abnormal pulse	A bradycardia (less than 60/min in adults), a tachycardia (more than 100/min in adults) or an irregular rhythm. Age-appropriate definitions of bradycardia and tachycardia should be used in children
New neurological deficit less than 24 hrs old	Any loss of neurological function that has come on within the previous 24 hours. This might include altered or lost sensation, weakness of the limbs (either transiently or permanently) and alterations in bladder or bowel function
Significant mechanism of injury	Penetrating injuries (stab or gunshot) and injuries with high energy transfer
Possible sepsis	Suspected sepsis in patients who present with altered mental state, low blood pressure (systolic less than 100) or raised respiratory rate (rate more than 22). In children, age specific physiological tools should be used to determine if possibly septic
New neurological deficit more than 24 hrs old	Any loss of neurological function including altered or lost sensation, weakness of the limbs (either transiently or permanently) and alterations in bladder or bowel function
Gross deformity	This will always be subjective. Gross and abnormal angulation or rotation is implied
Open fracture	All wounds in the vicinity of a fracture should be regarded with suspicion. If there is any possibility of communication between the wound and the fracture, then the fracture should be assumed to be open
Inappropriate history	When the history (story) given does not explain the physical findings it is termed inappropriate. This is important as it is a marker of safeguarding concerns in both adults and children
Deformity	This will always be subjective. Abnormal angulation or rotation is implied
Swelling	An abnormal increase in size

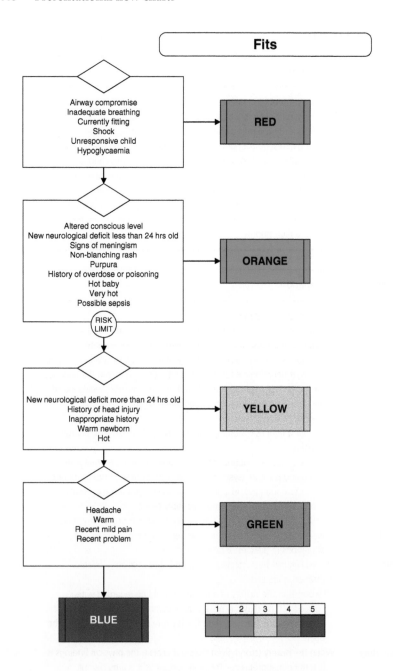

Notes accompanying fits

See also	Chart notes
Head injury Headache Overdose and poisoning	This is a presentation defined flow diagram. It is not an uncommon presentation to the Emergency Department and this chart is designed to allow rapid categorisation of patients who are currently fitting or who have fitted. A number of general discriminators are used including *Life threat*, *Conscious level* and *Temperature*. Specific discriminators include *Signs of meningism* and a focal or progressive loss of function. As with all unconscious patients rapid blood sugar estimation would be indicated to exclude hypoglycaemia

Specific discriminators	Explanation
Currently fitting	Patients who are in the tonic or clonic stages of a grand mal convulsion and patients currently experiencing partial fits
Hypoglycaemia	Glucose less than 3 mmol/l
New neurological deficit less than 24 hrs old	Any loss of neurological function that has come on within the previous 24 hours. This might include altered or lost sensation, weakness of the limbs (either transiently or permanently) and alterations in bladder or bowel function
Signs of meningism	Classically a stiff neck together with headache and photophobia
Non-blanching rash	A rash that does not blanch (go white) when pressure is applied to it. Often tested using a glass tumbler to apply pressure as any colour change can be observed through the bottom of the tumbler
Purpura	A rash on any part of the body that is caused by small haemorrhages under the skin. A purpuric rash does not blanch (go white) when pressure is applied to it
History of overdose or poisoning	This information may come from others or may be deduced if medication is missing
Possible sepsis	Suspected sepsis in patients who present with altered mental state, low blood pressure (systolic less than 100) or raised respiratory rate (rate more than 22). In children, age specific physiological tools should be used to determine if possibly septic
New neurological deficit more than 24 hrs old	Any loss of neurological function including altered or lost sensation, weakness of the limbs (either transiently or permanently) and alterations in bladder or bowel function
History of head injury	A history of a recent physically traumatic event involving the head. Usually this will be reported by the patient but if the patient has been unconscious this history should be sought from a reliable witness
Inappropriate history	When the history (story) given does not explain the physical findings it is termed inappropriate. This is important as it is a marker of safeguarding concerns in both adults and children
Headache	Any pain around the head that is not related to a particular anatomical structure. Facial pain is not included

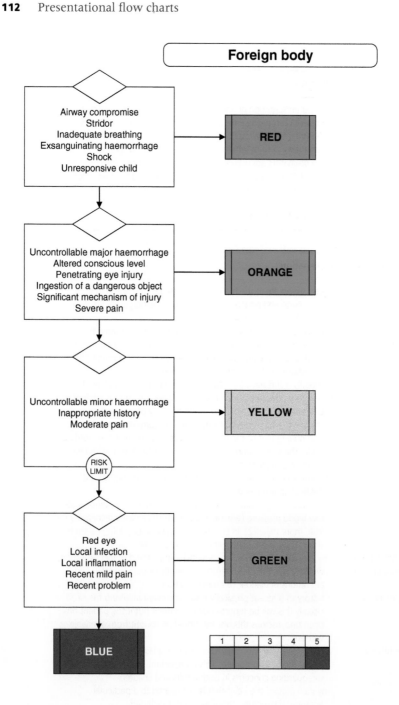

Foreign body

Airway compromise
Stridor
Inadequate breathing
Exsanguinating haemorrhage
Shock
Unresponsive child

RED

Uncontrollable major haemorrhage
Altered conscious level
Penetrating eye injury
Ingestion of a dangerous object
Significant mechanism of injury
Severe pain

ORANGE

Uncontrollable minor haemorrhage
Inappropriate history
Moderate pain

YELLOW

RISK
LIMIT

Red eye
Local infection
Local inflammation
Recent mild pain
Recent problem

GREEN

BLUE

| 1 | 2 | 3 | 4 | 5 |

Notes accompanying foreign body

See also	Chart notes
Torso injury Wounds	This is a presentation defined flow diagram designed to allow accurate prioritisation of patients who present with foreign bodies in any part of their anatomy. The severity of such cases can range from the inconvenient to the life threatening and this chart is designed to differentiate between these. A number of general discriminators have been used including *Life threat*, *Haemorrhage* and *Pain*. The only specific discriminator that relates to anatomical site is that of *Penetrating eye injury*

Specific discriminators	Explanation
Stridor	This may be an inspiratory or expiratory noise, or both. Stridor is heard best on breathing with the mouth open
Penetrating eye injury	A recent physically traumatic event involving penetration of the globe
Ingestion of a dangerous object	Ingestion of a dangerous or potentially dangerous foreign object e.g. button battery, magnets or razor blades which may be a potential threat to life
Significant mechanism of injury	Penetrating injuries (stab or gunshot) and injuries with high energy transfer
Inappropriate history	When the history (story) given does not explain the physical findings it is termed inappropriate. This is important as it is a marker of safeguarding concerns in both adults and children
Red eye	Any redness to the eye. A red eye may be painful or painless and may be complete or partial
Local infection	Local infection usually manifests as inflammation (pain, swelling and redness) confined to a particular site or area, with or without a collection of pus
Local inflammation	Local inflammation will involve pain, swelling and redness confined to a particular site or area

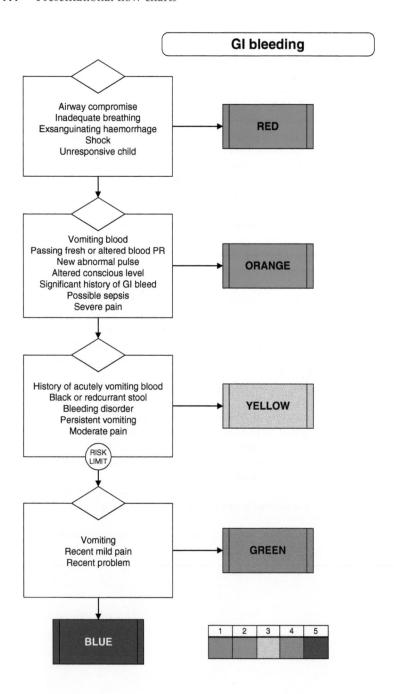

GI bleeding

Airway compromise
Inadequate breathing
Exsanguinating haemorrhage
Shock
Unresponsive child

RED

Vomiting blood
Passing fresh or altered blood PR
New abnormal pulse
Altered conscious level
Significant history of GI bleed
Possible sepsis
Severe pain

ORANGE

History of acutely vomiting blood
Black or redcurrant stool
Bleeding disorder
Persistent vomiting
Moderate pain

YELLOW

RISK
LIMIT

Vomiting
Recent mild pain
Recent problem

GREEN

BLUE

| 1 | 2 | 3 | 4 | 5 |

Notes accompanying GI bleeding

See also	Chart notes
Abdominal pain in adults Abdominal pain in children Diarrhoea and vomiting	This is a presentation defined flow diagram. Patients may present with GI bleeding either as vomiting altered or unaltered blood, or by passing blood PR. A number of general discriminators are used including *Life threat* and *Pain*. Specific discriminators have been selected to indicate the current severity of the GI bleeding. Thus patients vomiting blood or those passing fresh or altered blood PR have a higher category than those with a history of vomiting

Specific discriminators	Explanation
Vomiting blood	Vomited blood may be fresh (bright or dark red) or coffee ground in appearance
Passing fresh or altered blood PR	In active massive GI bleeding dark red blood will be passed PR. As GI transit time increases this becomes darker, eventually becoming melaena
Significant history of GI bleed	Any history of massive GI bleeding or of any GI bleed associated with oesophageal varices
Possible sepsis	Suspected sepsis in patients who present with altered mental state, low blood pressure (systolic less than 100) or raised respiratory rate (rate more than 22). In children, age specific physiological tools should be used to determine if possibly septic
History of acutely vomiting blood	Frank haematemesis, vomiting of altered blood (coffee ground) or of blood mixed in the vomit within the past 24 hours
Black or redcurrant stool	Any blackness fulfils the criteria of black stool while a dark red stool, classically seen in intussusceptions, is redcurrant stool
Bleeding disorder	Congenital or acquired bleeding disorder
Persistent vomiting	Vomiting that is continuous or that occurs without any respite between episodes
Vomiting	Any emesis

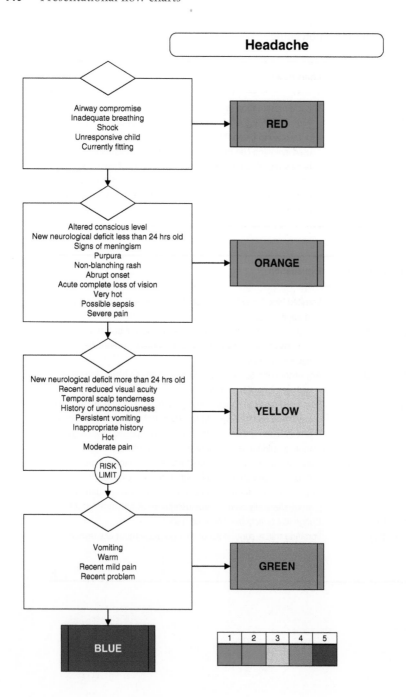

Headache

Airway compromise
Inadequate breathing
Shock
Unresponsive child
Currently fitting

RED

Altered conscious level
New neurological deficit less than 24 hrs old
Signs of meningism
Purpura
Non-blanching rash
Abrupt onset
Acute complete loss of vision
Very hot
Possible sepsis
Severe pain

ORANGE

New neurological deficit more than 24 hrs old
Recent reduced visual acuity
Temporal scalp tenderness
History of unconsciousness
Persistent vomiting
Inappropriate history
Hot
Moderate pain

YELLOW

RISK LIMIT

Vomiting
Warm
Recent mild pain
Recent problem

GREEN

BLUE

| 1 | 2 | 3 | 4 | 5 |

Notes accompanying headache

See also	Chart notes
Head injury Neck pain	This is a presentation defined flow diagram. A large number of conditions can present with headache and a number of these require urgent intervention. A number of general discriminators are used including *Life threat*, *Conscious level*, *Pain* and *Temperature*. Specific discriminators have been used to identify severe causes such as subarachnoid haemorrhage and meningococcaemia. New neurological signs or symptoms together with reduction in visual acuity and tenderness of the scalp are used to indicate the need for urgent clinical review

Specific discriminators	Explanation
New neurological deficit less than 24 hrs old	Any loss of neurological function that has come on within the previous 24 hours. This might include altered or lost sensation, weakness of the limbs (either transiently or permanently) and alterations in bladder or bowel function
Signs of meningism	Classically a stiff neck together with headache and photophobia
Purpura	A rash on any part of the body that is caused by small haemorrhages under the skin. A purpuric rash does not blanch (go white) when pressure is applied to it
Non-blanching rash	A rash that does not blanch (go white) when pressure is applied to it. Often tested using a glass tumbler to apply pressure as any colour change can be observed through the bottom of the tumbler
Abrupt onset	Onset within seconds or minutes. May cause waking from sleep
Acute complete loss of vision	Loss of vision in one or both eyes within the preceding 24 hours that has not returned to normal
Possible sepsis	Suspected sepsis in patients who present with altered mental state, low blood pressure (systolic less than 100) or raised respiratory rate (rate more than 22). In children, age specific physiological tools should be used to determine if possibly septic
New neurological deficit more than 24 hrs old	Any loss of neurological function including altered or lost sensation, weakness of the limbs (either transiently or permanently) and alterations in bladder or bowel function
Recent reduced visual acuity	Any reduction in corrected visual acuity within the past 7 days
Temporal scalp tenderness	Tenderness on palpation over the temporal area (especially over the artery)
History of unconsciousness	There may be a reliable witness who can state whether the patient was unconscious (and for how long). If not, a patient who is unable to remember the incident should be assumed to have been unconscious
Persistent vomiting	Vomiting that is continuous or that occurs without any respite between episodes
Inappropriate history	When the history (story) given does not explain the physical findings it is termed inappropriate. This is important as it is a marker of safeguarding concerns in both adults and children
Vomiting	Any emesis

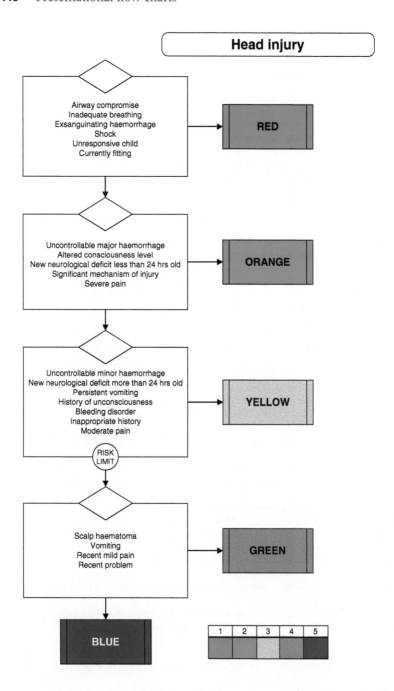

Head injury

Airway compromise
Inadequate breathing
Exsanguinating haemorrhage
Shock
Unresponsive child
Currently fitting

RED

Uncontrollable major haemorrhage
Altered consciousness level
New neurological deficit less than 24 hrs old
Significant mechanism of injury
Severe pain

ORANGE

Uncontrollable minor haemorrhage
New neurological deficit more than 24 hrs old
Persistent vomiting
History of unconsciousness
Bleeding disorder
Inappropriate history
Moderate pain

YELLOW

RISK
LIMIT

Scalp haematoma
Vomiting
Recent mild pain
Recent problem

GREEN

BLUE

1	2	3	4	5

Notes accompanying head injury

See also	Chart notes
Fits Headache Neck pain	This is a presentation defined flow diagram. Head injury is an extremely common presentation and its effects may vary from life-threatening extradural haemorrhage to minimal scalp injury. A number of general discriminators have been used including *Life threat, Conscious level (both in adults and children), Haemorrhage* and *Pain.* Specific discriminators are included to select those patients with significant mechanism and the development of neurological signs and symptoms to a higher priority

Specific discriminators	Explanation
Currently fitting	Patients who are in the tonic or clonic stages of a grand mal convulsion and patients currently experiencing partial fits
New neurological deficit less than 24 hrs old	Any loss of neurological function that has come on within the previous 24 hours. This might include altered or lost sensation, weakness of the limbs (either transiently or permanently) and alterations in bladder or bowel function
Significant mechanism of injury	Penetrating injuries (stab or gunshot) and injuries with high energy transfer
New neurological deficit more than 24 hrs old	Any loss of neurological function including altered or lost sensation, weakness of the limbs (either transiently or permanently) and alterations in bladder or bowel function
Persistent vomiting	Vomiting that is continuous or that occurs without any respite between episodes
History of unconsciousness	There may be a reliable witness who can state whether the patient was unconscious (and for how long). If not, a patient who is unable to remember the incident should be assumed to have been unconscious
Bleeding disorder	Congenital or acquired bleeding disorder
Inappropriate history	When the history (story) given does not explain the physical findings it is termed inappropriate. This is important as it is a marker of safeguarding concerns in both adults and children
Scalp haematoma	A raised bruised area to the scalp (bruises below the hair line at the front are to the forehead)
Vomiting	Any emesis

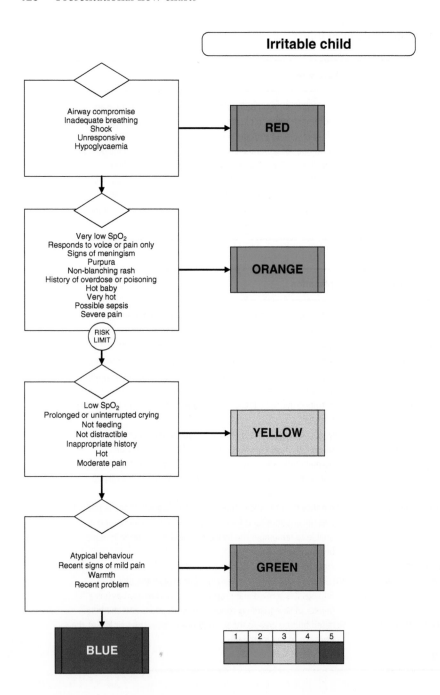

Irritable child

Airway compromise
Inadequate breathing
Shock
Unresponsive
Hypoglycaemia

RED

Very low SpO$_2$
Responds to voice or pain only
Signs of meningism
Purpura
Non-blanching rash
History of overdose or poisoning
Hot baby
Very hot
Possible sepsis
Severe pain

ORANGE

RISK LIMIT

Low SpO$_2$
Prolonged or uninterrupted crying
Not feeding
Not distractible
Inappropriate history
Hot
Moderate pain

YELLOW

Atypical behaviour
Recent signs of mild pain
Warmth
Recent problem

GREEN

BLUE

| 1 | 2 | 3 | 4 | 5 |

Notes accompanying irritable child

See also	Chart notes
Crying baby Unwell child Unwell newborn Worried parent	This is a presentation defined flow diagram. **It is designed to be used in children over the age of 12 months.** A number of general discriminators have been used including *Life threat*, *Conscious level* and *Pain*. Specific discriminators include those that allow recognition of more specific pathologies such as septicaemia, or which indicate that a more serious pathology might exist. The risk limit sits between ORANGE and YELLOW and therefore no children can be categorised as YELLOW, GREEN or BLUE until all the specific and general discriminators outlined under the RED and ORANGE categories have been specifically excluded. This may take longer than the time available for initial assessment. If the patient is under 28 days, the Unwell Newborn chart should be used

Specific discriminators	Explanation
Hypoglycaemia	Glucose less than 3 mmol/l
Very low SpO$_2$	This is a saturation of less than 95% on O$_2$ therapy or less than 92% on air
Signs of meningism	Classically a stiff neck together with headache and photophobia
Purpura	A rash on any part of the body that is caused by small haemorrhages under the skin. A purpuric rash does not blanch (go white) when pressure is applied to it
Non-blanching rash	A rash that does not blanch (go white) when pressure is applied to it. Often tested using a glass tumbler to apply pressure as any colour change can be observed through the bottom of the tumbler
History of overdose or poisoning	This information may come from others or may be deduced if medication is missing
Possible sepsis	Suspected sepsis in patients who present with altered mental state, low blood pressure (systolic less than 100) or raised respiratory rate (rate more than 22). In children, age specific physiological tools should be used to determine if possibly septic
Signs of severe pain	Young children and babies in severe pain cannot complain. They will usually cry out continuously and inconsolably and be tachycardic. They may well exhibit signs such as pallor and sweating
Low SpO$_2$	This is a saturation of less than 95% on air
Prolonged or uninterrupted crying	A child who has cried continuously for 2 hours or more
Not feeding	Children who will not take any solid or liquid (as appropriate) by mouth. Children who will take the food but always vomit afterwards may also fulfil this criterion
Not distractible	Children who are distressed by pain or other things who cannot be distracted by conversation or play
Inappropriate history	When the history (story) given does not explain the physical findings it is termed inappropriate. This is important as it is a marker of safeguarding concerns in both adults and children
Signs of moderate pain	Young children and babies in moderate pain cannot complain. They will usually cry intermittently and are often intermittently consolable
Atypical behaviour	Children who are behaving in a way that is not usual in the given situation. The carers will often volunteer this information. Such children are often referred to as fractious or 'out of sorts'

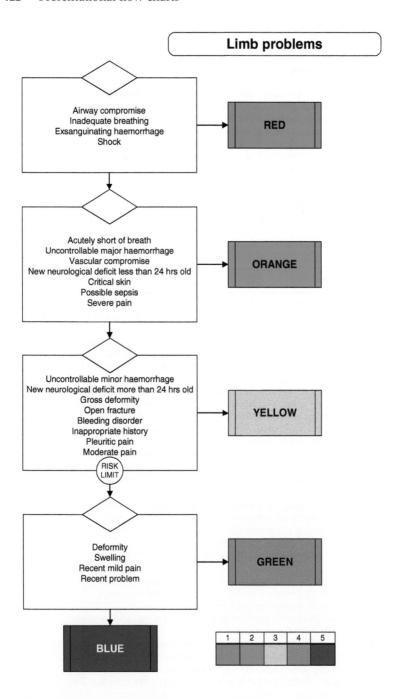

Notes accompanying limb problems

See also	Chart notes
Limping child	This is a presentation defined flow diagram. Injuries to the limbs are the commonest presentation to Emergency Departments and, while rarely life-threatening, may cause considerable morbidity. A number of general discriminators are used including *Life threat*, *Haemorrhage* and *Pain*. Specific discriminators are included to ensure that limb-threatening injuries are seen and treated urgently. Discriminators are also included to remind the triage practitioner to consider the signs and symptoms of thromboembolic disease and its complications

Specific discriminators	Explanation
Acutely short of breath	Shortness of breath that comes on suddenly, or a sudden exacerbation of chronic shortness of breath
Vascular compromise	There will be a combination of pallor, coldness, altered sensation and pain with or without absent pulses distal to the injury
New neurological deficit less than 24 hrs old	Any loss of neurological function that has come on within the previous 24 hours. This might include altered or lost sensation, weakness of the limbs (either transiently or permanently) and alterations in bladder or bowel function
Critical skin	A fracture or dislocation may leave fragments or ends of bone pressing so hard against the skin that the viability of the skin is threatened. The skin will be white and under tension
Possible sepsis	Suspected sepsis in patients who present with altered mental state, low blood pressure (systolic less than 100) or raised respiratory rate (rate more than 22). In children, age specific physiological tools should be used to determine if possibly septic
New neurological deficit more than 24 hrs old	Any loss of neurological function including altered or lost sensation, weakness of the limbs (either transiently or permanently) and alterations in bladder or bowel function
Gross deformity	This will always be subjective. Gross and abnormal angulation or rotation is implied
Open fracture	All wounds in the vicinity of a fracture should be regarded with suspicion. If there is any possibility of communication between the wound and the fracture, then the fracture should be assumed to be open
Bleeding disorder	Congenital or acquired bleeding disorder
Inappropriate history	When the history (story) given does not explain the physical findings it is termed inappropriate. This is important as it is a marker of safeguarding concerns in both adults and children
Pleuritic pain	A sharp, localised pain in the chest that worsens on breathing, coughing or sneezing
Deformity	This will always be subjective. Abnormal angulation or rotation is implied
Swelling	An abnormal increase in size

Limping child

Airway compromise
Inadequate breathing
Shock

RED

Vascular compromise
Purpura
Non-blanching rash
Hot baby
Very hot
Possible sepsis
Severe pain

RISK
LIMIT

ORANGE

Hot joint
Pain on joint movement
Bleeding disorder
Inappropriate history
Hot
Moderate pain

YELLOW

Deformity
Swelling
Warm
Recent mild pain
Recent problem

GREEN

BLUE

1	2	3	4	5

Notes accompanying limping child

See also	Chart notes
Limb problems	This is a presentation defined flow diagram. Children who present with limp range from those who have suffered a minor soft tissue injury to the foot or ankle to those who have developed septic arthritis of the hip. This chart is designed to allow accurate prioritisation of such children. A number of general discriminators are used including *Life threat*, *Pain* and *Temperature.* Specific discriminators have been included to allow children with more urgent pathologies that threaten distal function to be accurately identified, and to spot quickly those in whom the limp is a sinister sign of systemic disease. The risk limit sits between ORANGE and YELLOW and therefore no children can be categorised as YELLOW, GREEN or BLUE until all the specific and general discriminators outlined under the RED and ORANGE categories have been specifically excluded. This may take longer than the time available for initial assessment

Specific discriminators	Explanation
Vascular compromise	There will be a combination of pallor, coldness, altered sensation and pain with or without absent pulses distal to the injury
Purpura	A rash on any part of the body that is caused by small haemorrhages under the skin. A purpuric rash does not blanch (go white) when pressure is applied to it
Non-blanching rash	A rash that does not blanch (go white) when pressure is applied to it. Often tested using a glass tumbler to apply pressure as any colour change can be observed through the bottom of the tumbler
Possible sepsis	Suspected sepsis in patients who present with altered mental state, low blood pressure (systolic less than 100) or raised respiratory rate (rate more than 22). In children, age specific physiological tools should be used to determine if possibly septic
Hot joint	Any warmth around a joint. Often accompanied by redness
Pain on joint movement	This can be pain on either active (patient) movement or passive (examiner) movement
Bleeding disorder	Congenital or acquired bleeding disorder
Inappropriate history	When the history (story) given does not explain the physical findings it is termed inappropriate. This is important as it is a marker of safeguarding concerns in both adults and children
Deformity	This will always be subjective. Abnormal angulation or rotation is implied
Swelling	An abnormal increase in size

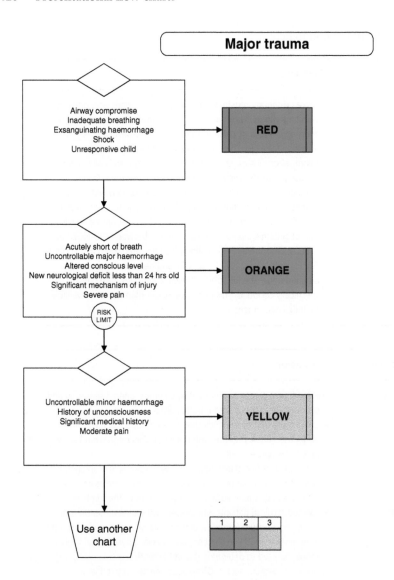

Major trauma

Airway compromise
Inadequate breathing
Exsanguinating haemorrhage
Shock
Unresponsive child

RED

Acutely short of breath
Uncontrollable major haemorrhage
Altered conscious level
New neurological deficit less than 24 hrs old
Significant mechanism of injury
Severe pain

ORANGE

RISK
LIMIT

Uncontrollable minor haemorrhage
History of unconsciousness
Significant medical history
Moderate pain

YELLOW

Use another
chart

1	2	3

Notes accompanying major trauma

See also	Chart notes
	Most health care providers know what is implied by major trauma but it is a strange presentation in that it is defined not by the patients or their injuries, but on some judgement of that injury by the carers. For this reason it is impossible to categorise a patient with this presentation as less than urgent. If it is necessary to do this, then a deliberate decision needs to be made that the original description of the patient as having suffered major trauma was incorrect, and the patient should be categorised using a different presentational flow diagram. A number of general discriminators have been used including *Life threat, Haemorrhage, Conscious level (both adult and child)* and *Pain.* Specific discriminators are designed to ensure that patients with a significant mechanism of injury are given a high enough urgency, and that those with pre-existing medical conditions and/or the development of new neurological signs are seen in good time

Specific discriminators	Explanation
Acutely short of breath	Shortness of breath that comes on suddenly, or a sudden exacerbation of chronic shortness of breath
New neurological deficit less than 24 hrs old	Any loss of neurological function that has come on within the previous 24 hours. This might include altered or lost sensation, weakness of the limbs (either transiently or permanently) and alterations in bladder or bowel function
Significant mechanism of injury	Penetrating injuries (stab or gunshot) and injuries with high energy transfer
History of unconsciousness	There may be a reliable witness who can state whether the patient was unconscious (and for how long). If not, a patient who is unable to remember the incident should be assumed to have been unconscious
Significant medical history	Any pre-existing medical condition requiring continual medication or other care

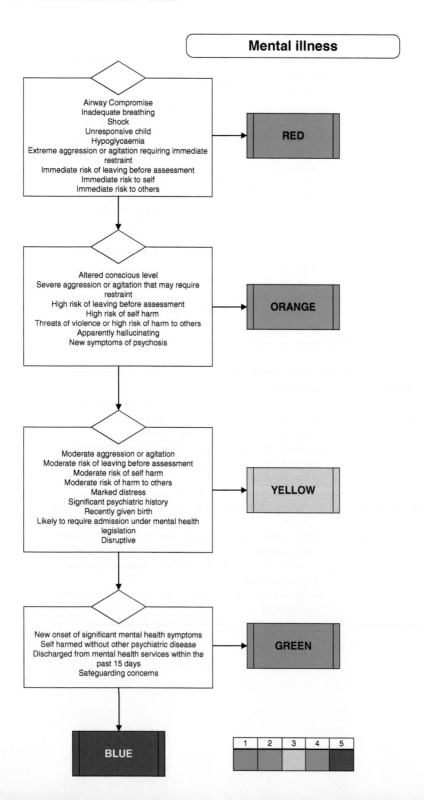

Notes accompanying mental illness

See also	Chart notes
Apparently drunk Behaving strangely	This is a presentation defined flow diagram that has been designed to allow clinical prioritisation of patients who present with known or newly declared mental illness. This includes patients who attended with a chief complaint which would indicate mental illness. A number of general discriminators have been used including *Life threat* and *Conscious level*. This chart is designed to allow assessment of both physical and psychiatric aspects of the presentation. Specific discriminators are included to allow accurate prioritisation of patients with a known significant psychiatric history and those who have varying degrees of risk of causing harm to others or to themselves. Patients who are disruptive or who are suffering severe distress are placed in the urgent category

Specific discriminators	Explanation
Hypoglycaemia	Glucose less than 3 mmol/l
High risk of self harm	An initial view of the risk of harm to self can be formed by considering the patient's behaviour. Patients who are threatening to harm themselves and who are actively seeking the means to do so are at high risk
Moderate risk of self harm	An initial view of the risk of harm to self can be formed by considering the patient's behaviour. Patients without a significant history of self harm, who are not actively trying to harm themselves, but who profess the desire to harm themselves are at moderate risk
Moderate risk of harm to others	An initial view of the risk of harm to others can be judged by looking at posture (tense, clenched), speech (loud, using threatening words) and motor behaviour (restless, pacing, lunging at others). Moderate risk should be assumed if there is any indication of potential harm to others
Marked distress	Patients who are markedly physically or emotionally upset
Significant psychiatric history	A history of a major psychiatric illness or event
Likely to require admission under mental health legislation	Patients with significant psychiatric symptoms who are likely to require admission under mental health legislation
Disruptive	Disruptive behaviour is behaviour that affects the smooth running of the department. It may be threatening

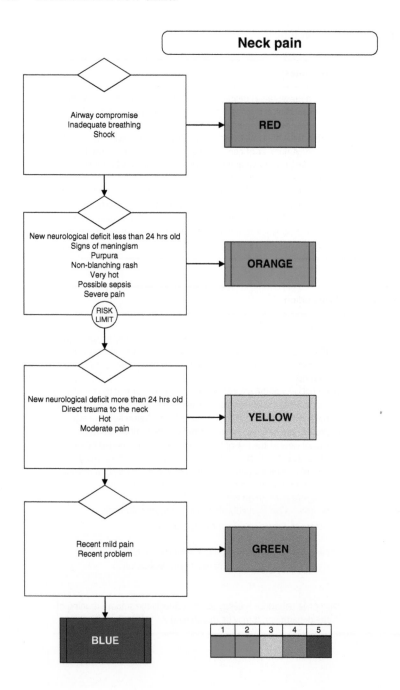

Neck pain

Airway compromise
Inadequate breathing
Shock

RED

New neurological deficit less than 24 hrs old
Signs of meningism
Purpura
Non-blanching rash
Very hot
Possible sepsis
Severe pain

RISK
LIMIT

ORANGE

New neurological deficit more than 24 hrs old
Direct trauma to the neck
Hot
Moderate pain

YELLOW

Recent mild pain
Recent problem

GREEN

BLUE

1	2	3	4	5

Notes accompanying neck pain

See also	Chart notes
Back pain Headache	This is a presentation defined flow diagram. Pain in the neck may arise because of local pathology or meningeal irritation. This chart is designed to allow rapid identification of patients presenting with symptoms or signs that indicate more urgent pathologies. A number of general discriminators are used including *Life threat*, *Pain* and *Temperature*. The specific discriminators that indicate meningitis are included under the ORANGE category

Specific discriminators	Explanation
New neurological deficit less than 24 hrs old	Any loss of neurological function that has come on within the previous 24 hours. This might include altered or lost sensation, weakness of the limbs (either transiently or permanently) and alterations in bladder or bowel function
Signs of meningism	Classically a stiff neck together with headache and photophobia
Purpura	A rash on any part of the body that is caused by small haemorrhages under the skin. A purpuric rash does not blanch (go white) when pressure is applied to it
Non-blanching rash	A rash that does not blanch (go white) when pressure is applied to it. Often tested using a glass tumbler to apply pressure as any colour change can be observed through the bottom of the tumbler
Possible sepsis	Suspected sepsis in patients who present with altered mental state, low blood pressure (systolic less than 100) or raised respiratory rate (rate more than 22). In children, age specific physiological tools should be used to determine if possibly septic
New neurological deficit more than 24 hrs old	Any loss of neurological function including altered or lost sensation, weakness of the limbs (either transiently or permanently) and alterations in bladder or bowel function
Direct trauma to the neck	This may be top to bottom (loading), for instance when something falls on the head, bending (forwards, backwards or to the side), twisting or distracting such as in hanging

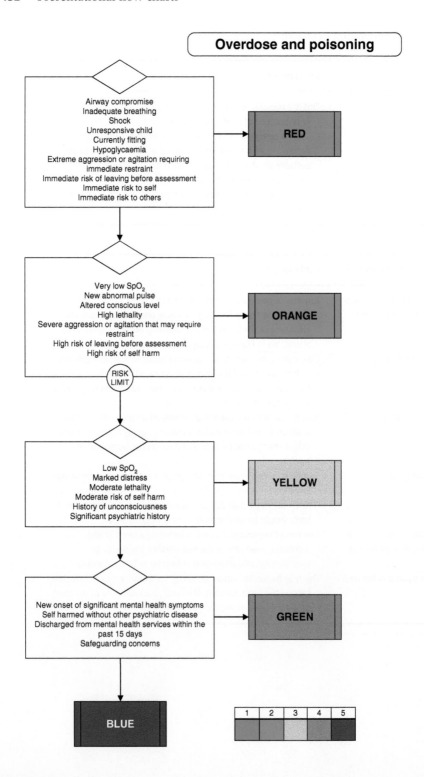

Overdose and poisoning

Airway compromise
Inadequate breathing
Shock
Unresponsive child
Currently fitting
Hypoglycaemia
Extreme aggression or agitation requiring
immediate restraint
Immediate risk of leaving before assessment
Immediate risk to self
Immediate risk to others

RED

Very low SpO$_2$
New abnormal pulse
Altered conscious level
High lethality
Severe aggression or agitation that may require
restraint
High risk of leaving before assessment
High risk of self harm

ORANGE

RISK
LIMIT

Low SpO$_2$
Marked distress
Moderate lethality
Moderate risk of self harm
History of unconsciousness
Significant psychiatric history

YELLOW

New onset of significant mental health symptoms
Self harmed without other psychiatric disease
Discharged from mental health services within the
past 15 days
Safeguarding concerns

GREEN

BLUE

| 1 | 2 | 3 | 4 | 5 |

Notes accompanying overdose and poisoning

See also	Chart notes
Self-harm	This is a presentation defined flow diagram. The flow chart has been designed to allow both the physical and psychiatric aspects of overdose to be considered, and to ensure accurate prioritisation of patients from both perspectives. It also allows prioritisation of patients who have been accidentally (or deliberately) poisoned by others. A number of general discriminators have been used including *Life threat* and *Unconscious level (in both children and adults)*. Specific discriminators include the assessed lethality of the overdose (which can be decided following discussion with a poisons centre) and an assessment of the risk of further attempts at self-harm

Specific discriminators	Explanation
Hypoglycaemia	Glucose less than 3 mmol/l
Very low SpO$_2$	This is a saturation of less than 95% on O$_2$ therapy or less than 92% on air
New abnormal pulse	A bradycardia (less than 60/min in adults), a tachycardia (more than 100/min in adults) or an irregular rhythm. Age-appropriate definitions of bradycardia and tachycardia should be used in children
High lethality	Lethality is the potential of the substance taken to cause harm. Advice from a poisons centre may be required to establish the level of risk of serious illness or death. If in doubt, assume a high risk
High risk of self harm	An initial view of the risk of harm to self can be formed by considering the patient's behaviour. Patients who are threatening to harm themselves and who are actively seeking the means to do so are at high risk
Low SpO$_2$	This is a saturation of less than 95% on air
Marked distress	Patients who are markedly physically or emotionally upset
Moderate lethality	Lethality is the potential of the substance taken to cause serious illness or death. Advice from a poisons centre may be required to establish the level of risk to the patient
Moderate risk of self-harm	An initial view of the risk of harm to self can be formed by considering the patient's behaviour. Patients without a significant history of self harm, who are not actively trying to harm themselves, but who profess the desire to harm themselves are at moderate risk
History of unconsciousness	There may be a reliable witness who can state whether the patient was unconscious (and for how long). If not, a patient who is unable to remember the incident should be assumed to have been unconscious
Significant psychiatric history	A history of a major psychiatric illness or event

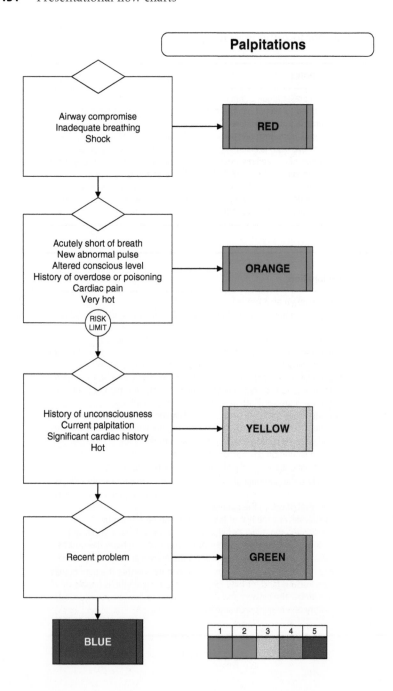

Notes accompanying palpitations

See also	Chart notes
Chest pain Collapse Unwell adult	This is a presentation defined flow diagram designed to allow the accurate prioritisation of those patients who present with a chief complaint of palpitations. Palpitations can have many causes ranging from the effects of ischaemic heart disease and other cardiac abnormalities to anxiety. Whatever the cause, it is their effect on circulation and their propensity to develop into life-threatening dysrhythmias that determine the clinical priority of the patient. Thus this chart is written to ensure that the signs and symptoms of cardiac insufficiency are included in the RED and ORANGE categories, together with historical pointers to potential early problems

Specific discriminators	Explanation
Acutely short of breath	Shortness of breath that comes on suddenly, or a sudden exacerbation of chronic shortness of breath
New abnormal pulse	A bradycardia (less than 60/min in adults), a tachycardia (more than 100/min in adults) or an irregular rhythm. Age-appropriate definitions of bradycardia and tachycardia should be used in children
History of overdose or poisoning	This information may come from others or may be deduced if medication is missing
Cardiac pain	Classically a severe dull 'gripping' or 'heavy' pain in the centre of the chest, radiating to the left arm or to the neck. May be associated with sweating and nausea
History of unconsciousness	There may be a reliable witness who can state whether the patient was unconscious (and for how long). If not, a patient who is unable to remember the incident should be assumed to have been unconscious
Current palpitation	A feeling of the heart racing (often described as a fluttering) that is still present
Significant cardiac history	A known recurrent dysrhythmia that has life-threatening effects is significant, as is a known cardiac condition which may deteriorate rapidly

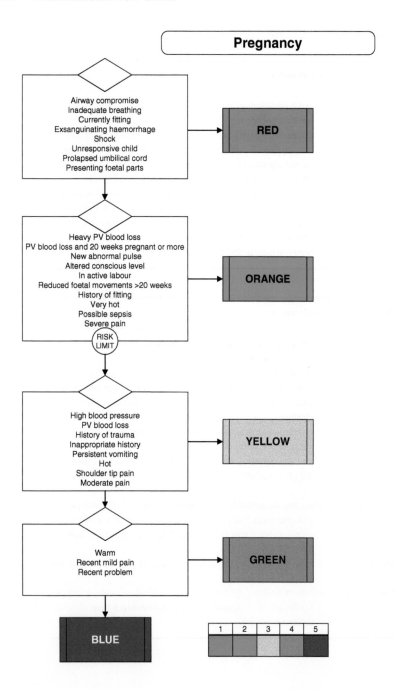

Pregnancy

Airway compromise
Inadequate breathing
Currently fitting
Exsanguinating haemorrhage
Shock
Unresponsive child
Prolapsed umbilical cord
Presenting foetal parts

RED

Heavy PV blood loss
PV blood loss and 20 weeks pregnant or more
New abnormal pulse
Altered conscious level
In active labour
Reduced foetal movements >20 weeks
History of fitting
Very hot
Possible sepsis
Severe pain

RISK LIMIT

ORANGE

High blood pressure
PV blood loss
History of trauma
Inappropriate history
Persistent vomiting
Hot
Shoulder tip pain
Moderate pain

YELLOW

Warm
Recent mild pain
Recent problem

GREEN

BLUE

1	2	3	4	5

Notes accompanying pregnancy

See also	Chart notes
PV bleeding	This is a presentation defined flow diagram. Pregnant women may attend the Emergency Department at all stages of pregnancy and with a variety of complaints. Some may be unaware of their pregnancy A number of general discriminators have been used including *Pain* and *Conscious level*. Specific discriminators are designed to allow early recognition of complications of pregnancy at all stages

Specific discriminators	Explanation
Prolapsed umbilical cord	Prolapse of any part of the umbilical cord through the cervix
Presenting foetal parts	Crowning or presentation of any other foetal part in the vagina
Heavy PV blood loss	PV loss is extremely difficult to assess. The presence of large clots or constant flow fulfils this criterion. The use of a large number of sanitary towels is suggestive of heavy loss
PV blood loss and 20 weeks pregnant or more	Any loss of blood PV in a woman known to be beyond the 20th week of pregnancy
New abnormal pulse	A bradycardia (less than 60/min in adults), a tachycardia (more then 100/min in adults) or an irregular rhythm. Age-appropriate definitions of bradycardia and tachycardia should be used in children
In active labour	A woman who is having regular and frequent painful contractions
Reduced foetal movements >20 weeks	Absent or reduced foetal movements during the previous 12 hours in a woman known to be beyond the 20th week of pregnancy
History of fitting	Any observed or reported fits that have occurred during the period of illness or following an episode of trauma
Possible sepsis	Suspected sepsis in patients who present with altered mental state, low blood pressure (systolic less than 100) or raised respiratory rate (rate more than 22). In children, age specific physiological tools should be used to determine if possibly septic
High blood pressure	A history of raised blood pressure or a raised blood pressure on examination
PV blood loss	Any loss of blood PV
History of trauma	A history of a recent physically traumatic event
Inappropriate history	When the history (story) given does not explain the physical findings it is termed inappropriate. This is important as it is a marker of safeguarding concerns in both adults and children
Persistent vomiting	Vomiting that is continuous or that occurs without any respite between episodes
Shoulder tip pain	Pain felt in the tip of the shoulder. This often indicates diaphragmatic irritation

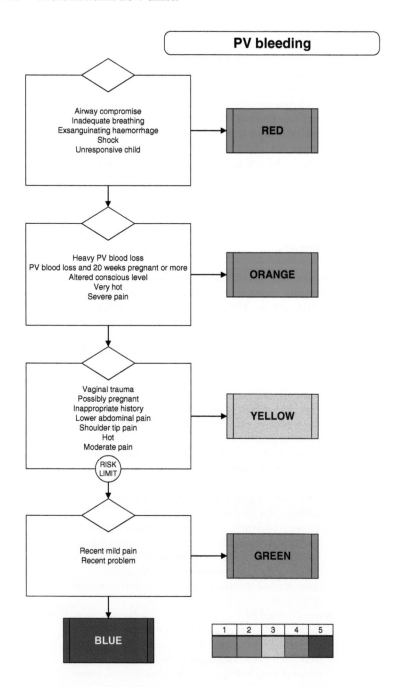

PV bleeding

Airway compromise
Inadequate breathing
Exsanguinating haemorrhage
Shock
Unresponsive child

RED

Heavy PV blood loss
PV blood loss and 20 weeks pregnant or more
Altered conscious level
Very hot
Severe pain

ORANGE

Vaginal trauma
Possibly pregnant
Inappropriate history
Lower abdominal pain
Shoulder tip pain
Hot
Moderate pain

YELLOW

RISK LIMIT

Recent mild pain
Recent problem

GREEN

BLUE

1	2	3	4	5

Notes accompanying PV bleeding

See also	Chart notes
Abdominal pain Pregnancy	This is a presentation defined flow diagram. PV bleeding may occur in pregnant and non-pregnant women and may have a large number of undefined causes. A number of general discriminators are used including *Life threat*, *Haemorrhage* and *Pain*

Specific discriminators	Explanation
Heavy PV blood loss	PV loss is extremely difficult to assess. The presence of large clots or constant flow fulfils this criterion. The use of a large number of sanitary towels is suggestive of heavy loss
PV blood loss and 20 weeks pregnant or more	Any loss of blood PV in a woman known to be beyond the 20th week of pregnancy
Vaginal trauma	Any history or other evidence of direct trauma to the vagina
Possibly pregnant	Any woman whose normal menstruation has failed to occur is possibly pregnant. Furthermore any woman of childbearing age who is having unprotected sex should be considered to be potentially pregnant
Inappropriate history	When the history (story) given does not explain the physical findings it is termed inappropriate. This is important as it is a marker of safeguarding concerns in both adults and children
Lower abdominal pain	Any pain felt in the lower abdomen. Abdominal pain associated with back pain may indicate abdominal aortic aneurysm, while association with PV bleeding may indicate ectopic pregnancy or miscarriage
Shoulder tip pain	Pain felt in the tip of the shoulder. This often indicates diaphragmatic irritation

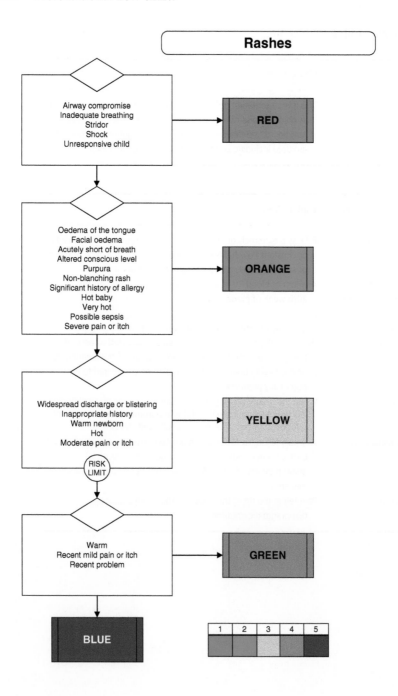

Rashes

Airway compromise
Inadequate breathing
Stridor
Shock
Unresponsive child

RED

Oedema of the tongue
Facial oedema
Acutely short of breath
Altered conscious level
Purpura
Non-blanching rash
Significant history of allergy
Hot baby
Very hot
Possible sepsis
Severe pain or itch

ORANGE

Widespread discharge or blistering
Inappropriate history
Warm newborn
Hot
Moderate pain or itch

YELLOW

RISK
LIMIT

Warm
Recent mild pain or itch
Recent problem

GREEN

BLUE

| 1 | 2 | 3 | 4 | 5 |

Notes accompanying rashes

See also	Chart notes
Allergy Bites and stings Unwell adult Unwell child	This is a presentation defined flow diagram. A rash may signify serious disease such as meningococcal septicaemia, or may be a sign of a chronic, non-acute problem such as psoriasis. Two general discriminators – *Life threat* and *Temperature* – are used in this chart. A larger number of specific discriminators are included in the ORANGE and YELLOW categories to ensure that more *serious* conditions are suitably triaged. In particular, purpura and associations of acute anaphylaxis appear at the ORANGE level

Specific discriminators	Explanation
Stridor	This may be an inspiratory or expiratory noise, or both. Stridor is heard best on breathing with the mouth open
Oedema of the tongue	Swelling of the tongue of any degree
Facial oedema	Diffuse swelling around the face, usually involving the lips
Acutely short of breath	Shortness of breath that comes on suddenly, or a sudden exacerbation of chronic shortness of breath
Purpura	A rash on any part of the body that is caused by small haemorrhages under the skin. A purpuric rash does not blanch (go white) when pressure is applied to it
Non-blanching rash	A rash that does not blanch (go white) when pressure is applied to it. Often tested using a glass tumbler to apply pressure as any colour change can be observed through the bottom of the tumbler
Significant history of allergy	A known sensitivity with severe reaction (e.g. to nuts or bee sting) is significant
Possible sepsis	Suspected sepsis in patients who present with altered mental state, low blood pressure (systolic less than 100) or raised respiratory rate (rate more than 22). In children, age specific physiological tools should be used to determine if possibly septic
Widespread discharge or blistering	Any discharging or blistering eruption covering more than 10% of the body surface area
Inappropriate history	When the history (story) given does not explain the physical findings it is termed inappropriate. This is important as it is a marker of safeguarding concerns in both adults and children

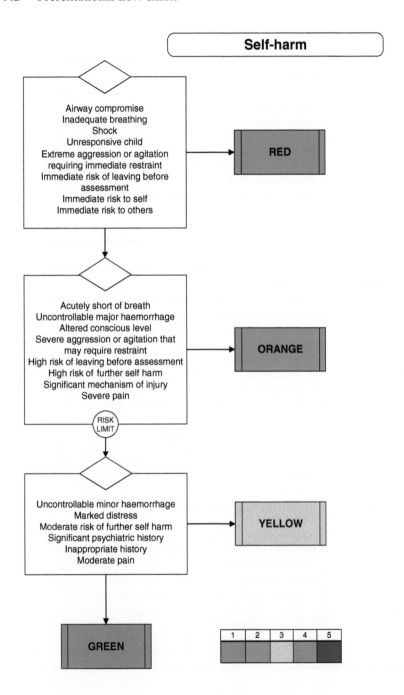

Notes accompanying self-harm

See also	Chart notes
Mental illness Overdose and poisoning	This is a presentation defined flow diagram. This flow diagram has been designed to allow accurate prioritisation of patients who have caused physical harm to themselves. This chart is designed to allow assessment of both physical and psychiatric aspects of the presentation. A separate chart entitled Overdose and poisoning has been designed as well. A number of general discriminators are used including *Life threat*, *Haemorrhage*, *Conscious level* and *Pain*. Specific discriminators are included to allow accurate prioritisation of patients with significant mechanisms of injury and those who have various degrees of risk of further self-harm

Specific discriminators	Explanation
Acutely short of breath	Shortness of breath that comes on suddenly, or a sudden exacerbation of chronic shortness of breath
High risk of further self harm	An initial view of the risk of harm to self can be formed by considering the patient's behaviour. Patients who are threatening to harm themselves and who are actively seeking the means to do so are at high risk
Significant mechanism of injury	Penetrating injuries (stab or gunshot) and injuries with high energy transfer
Marked distress	Patients who are markedly physically or emotionally upset
Moderate risk of further self-harm	An initial view of the risk of harm to self can be formed by considering the patient's behaviour. Patients without a significant history of self harm, who are not actively trying to harm themselves, but who profess the desire to harm themselves further are at moderate risk
Significant psychiatric history	A history of a major psychiatric illness or event
Inappropriate history	When the history (story) given does not explain the physical findings it is termed inappropriate. This is important as it is a marker of safeguarding concerns in both adults and children

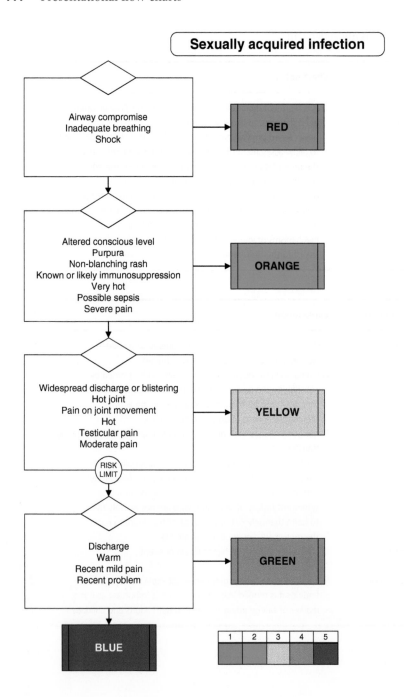

Sexually acquired infection

Airway compromise
Inadequate breathing
Shock

RED

Altered conscious level
Purpura
Non-blanching rash
Known or likely immunosuppression
Very hot
Possible sepsis
Severe pain

ORANGE

Widespread discharge or blistering
Hot joint
Pain on joint movement
Hot
Testicular pain
Moderate pain

YELLOW

RISK
LIMIT

Discharge
Warm
Recent mild pain
Recent problem

GREEN

BLUE

1	2	3	4	5

Notes accompanying sexually acquired infection

See also	Chart notes
	This is a presentation defined flow diagram which has been included to allow prioritisation of patients who attend with known or obvious sexual acquired infection. A number of general discriminators are used including *Life threat*, *Pain* and *Temperature*. Specific discriminators have been added to allow identification of more urgent conditions such as gonococcaemia. It is important to ensure that preconceptions about the disposal of these patients do not prevent appropriate triage

Specific discriminators	Explanation
Purpura	A rash on any part of the body that is caused by small haemorrhages under the skin. A purpuric rash does not blanch (go white) when pressure is applied to it
Non-blanching rash	A rash that does not blanch (go white) when pressure is applied to it. Often tested using a glass tumbler to apply pressure as any colour change can be observed through the bottom of the tumbler
Known or likely immunosuppression	Any patient who is known or likely to be immunosuppressed including those on immunosuppressive drugs (including long-term steroids)
Possible sepsis	Suspected sepsis in patients who present with altered mental state, low blood pressure (systolic less than 100) or raised respiratory rate (rate more than 22). In children, age specific physiological tools should be used to determine if possibly septic
Widespread discharge or blistering	Any discharging or blistering eruption covering more than 10% of the body surface area
Hot joint	Any warmth around a joint. Often accompanied by redness
Pain on joint movement	This can be pain on either active (patient) movement or passive (examiner) movement
Testicular pain	Pain in the testicles
Discharge	In the context of sexually acquired infection this is any discharge from the penis or abnormal discharge from the vagina

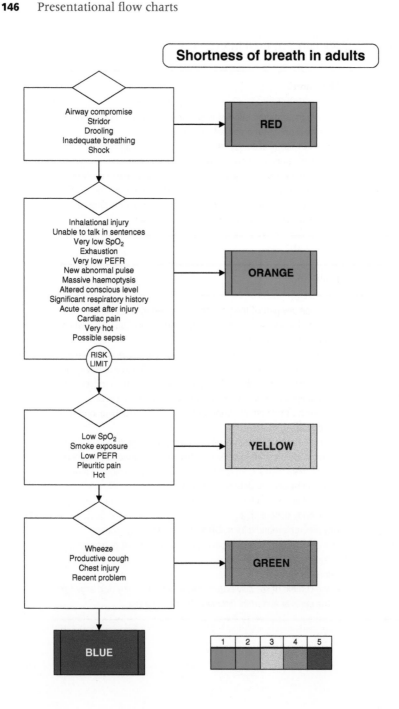

Shortness of breath in adults

Airway compromise
Stridor
Drooling
Inadequate breathing
Shock

RED

Inhalational injury
Unable to talk in sentences
Very low SpO$_2$
Exhaustion
Very low PEFR
New abnormal pulse
Massive haemoptysis
Altered conscious level
Significant respiratory history
Acute onset after injury
Cardiac pain
Very hot
Possible sepsis

RISK
LIMIT

ORANGE

Low SpO$_2$
Smoke exposure
Low PEFR
Pleuritic pain
Hot

YELLOW

Wheeze
Productive cough
Chest injury
Recent problem

GREEN

BLUE

| 1 | 2 | 3 | 4 | 5 |

Notes accompanying shortness of breath in adults

See also	Chart notes
Asthma Shortness of breath in children Unwell adult	This is a presentation defined flow diagram. Shortness of breath may be the presenting symptom for a number of cardiovascular and respiratory problems. A number of general discriminators are used including *Life threat* and *Oxygen saturation*. Specific discriminators include those which are present in severe asthma, COPD and ischaemic heart disease

Specific discriminators	Explanation
Stridor	This may be an inspiratory or expiratory noise, or both. Stridor is heard best on breathing with the mouth open
Drooling	Saliva running from the mouth as a result of being unable to swallow
Inhalational injury	A history of being confined in a smoke-filled space is the most reliable indicator of smoke inhalation. Carbon deposits around the mouth and nose and hoarse voice may be present. History is also the most reliable way of diagnosing inhalation of chemicals – there will not necessarily be any signs
Unable to talk in sentences	Patients who are so breathless that they cannot complete relatively short sentences in one breath
Very low SpO$_2$	This is a saturation of less than 95% on O$_2$ therapy or less than 92% on air
Exhaustion	Exhausted patients appear to reduce the effort they make to breathe despite continuing respiratory insufficiency. This is pre-terminal
Very low PEFR	The PEFR predicted after consideration of the age and sex of the patient. Some patients may know their 'best' PEFR and this may be used. If the ratio of measured to predicted is less than 33% then this criterion is fulfilled
New abnormal pulse	A bradycardia (less than 60/min in adults), a tachycardia (more than 100/min in adults) or an irregular rhythm. Age-appropriate definitions of bradycardia and tachycardia should be used in children
Massive haemoptysis	Coughing up large amounts of fresh or clotted blood. Not to be confused with streaks of blood in saliva
Significant respiratory history	A history of previous life-threatening episodes of a respiratory condition (e.g. COPD) is significant, as is brittle asthma
Acute onset after injury	Onset of symptoms immediately within 24 hours of a physically traumatic event
Cardiac pain	Classically a severe dull 'gripping' or 'heavy' pain in the centre of the chest, radiating to the left arm or to the neck. May be associated with sweating and nausea
Possible sepsis	Suspected sepsis in patients who present with altered mental state, low blood pressure (systolic less than 100) or raised respiratory rate (rate more than 22). In children, age specific physiological tools should be used to determine if possibly septic
Low SpO$_2$	This is a saturation of less than 95% on air
Smoke exposure	Smoke inhalation should be assumed if the patient has been confined in a smoke-filled space. Physical signs such as oral or nasal soot are less reliable but significant if present
Low PEFR	The PEFR predicted after consideration of the age and sex of the patient. Some patients may know their 'best' PEFR and this may be used. If the ratio of measured to predicted is less than 50% then this criterion is fulfilled
Pleuritic pain	A sharp, localised pain in the chest that worsens on breathing, coughing or sneezing
Wheeze	This can be audible wheeze or a feeling of wheeze. Very severe airway obstruction is silent (no air can move)
Productive cough	A cough that is productive of phlegm, whatever the colour
Chest injury	Any injury to the area below the clavicles and above the level of the lowest rib. Injury to the lower part of the chest can cause underlying damage to abdominal organs

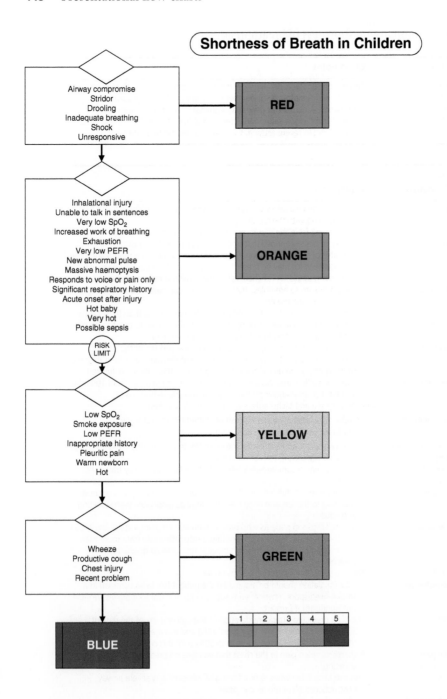

Shortness of Breath in Children

Airway compromise
Stridor
Drooling
Inadequate breathing
Shock
Unresponsive

RED

Inhalational injury
Unable to talk in sentences
Very low SpO$_2$
Increased work of breathing
Exhaustion
Very low PEFR
New abnormal pulse
Massive haemoptysis
Responds to voice or pain only
Significant respiratory history
Acute onset after injury
Hot baby
Very hot
Possible sepsis

ORANGE

RISK
LIMIT

Low SpO$_2$
Smoke exposure
Low PEFR
Inappropriate history
Pleuritic pain
Warm newborn
Hot

YELLOW

Wheeze
Productive cough
Chest injury
Recent problem

GREEN

BLUE

1	2	3	4	5

Notes accompanying shortness of breath in children

See also	Chart notes
Asthma Unwell child Unwell newborn	This is a presentation defined flow diagram that applies to children under the age of 14 years. A number of general discriminators are used including *Life threat* and *Oxygen saturation*. Specific discriminators have been included to allow accurate identification of children who are suffering the severe effects of asthma and those in whom there is more serious pathology. Accurate peak flow reading is difficult in young children and in such cases this discriminator should be ignored. Peak flow readings when obtained should always be related to the expected peak flow for age and sex. The risk limit sits between ORANGE and YELLOW and therefore no children can be categorised as YELLOW, GREEN or BLUE until all the specific and general discriminators outlined under the RED and ORANGE categories have been specifically excluded. This may take longer than the time available for initial assessment. If the patient is under 28 days, the Unwell Newborn chart should be used

Specific discriminators	Explanation
Stridor	This may be an inspiratory or expiratory noise, or both. Stridor is heard best on breathing with the mouth open
Drooling	Saliva running from the mouth as a result of being unable to swallow
Inhalational injury	A history of being confined in a smoke-filled space is the most reliable indicator of smoke inhalation. Carbon deposits around the mouth and nose and hoarse voice may be present. History is also the most reliable way of diagnosing inhalation of chemicals – there will not necessarily be any signs
Unable to talk in sentences	Patients who are so breathless that they cannot complete relatively short sentences in one breath
Very low SpO_2	This is a saturation of less than 95% on O_2 therapy or less than 92% on air
Increased work of breathing	Increased work of breathing is shown as increased respiratory rate, use of accessory muscles and grunting
Exhaustion	Exhausted patients appear to reduce the effort they make to breathe despite continuing respiratory insufficiency. This is pre-terminal
Very low PEFR	The PEFR predicted after consideration of the age and sex of the patient. Some patients may know their 'best' PEFR and this may be used. If the ratio of measured to predicted is less than 33% then this criterion is fulfilled
New abnormal pulse	A bradycardia (less than 60/min in adults), a tachycardia (more than 100/min in adults) or an irregular rhythm. Age-appropriate definitions of bradycardia and tachycardia should be used in children
Massive haemoptysis	Coughing up large amounts of fresh or clotted blood. Not to be confused with streaks of blood in saliva
Significant respiratory history	A history of previous life-threatening episodes of a respiratory condition (e.g. COPD) is significant, as is brittle asthma
Acute onset after injury	Onset of symptoms immediately within 24 hours of a physically traumatic event
Possible sepsis	Suspected sepsis in patients who present with altered mental state, low blood pressure (systolic less than 100) or raised respiratory rate (rate more than 22). In children, age specific physiological tools should be used to determine if possibly septic
Low SpO_2	This is a saturation of less than 95% on air
Smoke exposure	Smoke inhalation should be assumed if the patient has been confined in a smoke-filled space. Physical signs such as oral or nasal soot are less reliable but significant if present
Low PEFR	The PEFR predicted after consideration of the age and sex of the patient. Some patients may know their 'best' PEFR and this may be used. If the ratio of measured to predicted is less than 50% then this criterion is fulfilled
Inappropriate history	When the history (story) given does not explain the physical findings it is termed inappropriate. This is important as it is a marker of safeguarding concerns in both adults and children
Pleuritic pain	A sharp, localised pain in the chest that worsens on breathing, coughing or sneezing
Wheeze	This can be audible wheeze or a feeling of wheeze. Very severe airway obstruction is silent (no air can move)
Productive cough	A cough that is productive of phlegm, whatever the colour
Chest injury	Any injury to the area below the clavicles and above the level of the lowest rib. Injury to the lower part of the chest can cause underlying damage to abdominal organs

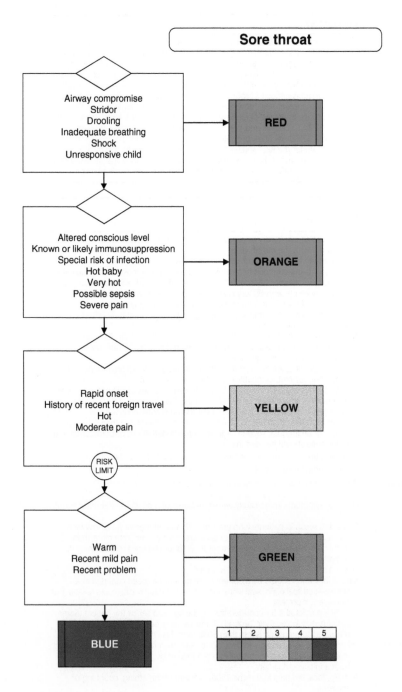

Sore throat

Airway compromise
Stridor
Drooling
Inadequate breathing
Shock
Unresponsive child

RED

Altered conscious level
Known or likely immunosuppression
Special risk of infection
Hot baby
Very hot
Possible sepsis
Severe pain

ORANGE

Rapid onset
History of recent foreign travel
Hot
Moderate pain

YELLOW

RISK
LIMIT

Warm
Recent mild pain
Recent problem

GREEN

BLUE

| 1 | 2 | 3 | 4 | 5 |

Notes accompanying sore throat

See also	Chart notes
Shortness of breath in adults Shortness of breath in children Unwell adult Unwell child Unwell newborn	This is a presentation defined flow diagram designed to allow accurate prioritisation for patients attending with sore throat. As problems with the throat can affect the airway there are a number of conditions that have this presentation and have a high priority. A number of general discriminators are used including *Life threat*, *Pain* and *Temperature*. Specific discriminators have been included to indicate where there is a high chance of more serious pathology. If the patient is under 28 days, the Unwell Newborn chart should be used

Specific discriminators	Explanation
Stridor	This may be an inspiratory or expiratory noise, or both. Stridor is heard best on breathing with the mouth open
Drooling	Saliva running from the mouth as a result of being unable to swallow
Known or likely immunosuppression	Any patient who is known or likely to be immunosuppressed including those on immunosuppressive drugs (including long-term steroids)
Special risk of infection	Known exposure to a dangerous pathogen, or travel to an area with an identified, current, serious infectious risk
Possible sepsis	Suspected sepsis in patients who present with altered mental state, low blood pressure (systolic less than 100) or raised respiratory rate (rate more than 22). In children, age specific physiological tools should be used to determine if possibly septic
Rapid onset	Onset within the preceding 12 hours
History of recent foreign travel	Recent significant foreign travel (within 2 weeks)

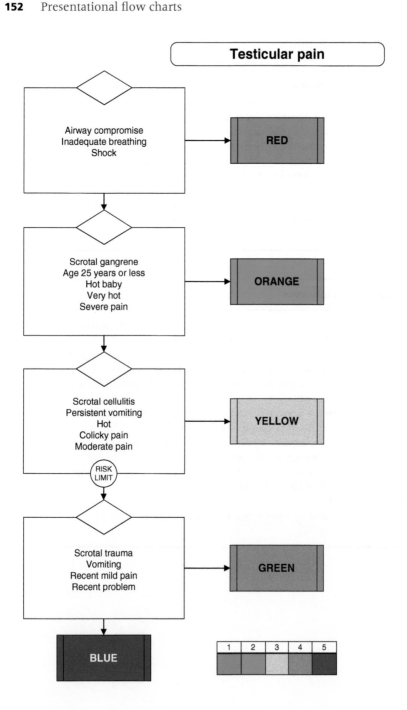

Testicular pain

Airway compromise
Inadequate breathing
Shock

RED

Scrotal gangrene
Age 25 years or less
Hot baby
Very hot
Severe pain

ORANGE

Scrotal cellulitis
Persistent vomiting
Hot
Colicky pain
Moderate pain

YELLOW

RISK
LIMIT

Scrotal trauma
Vomiting
Recent mild pain
Recent problem

GREEN

BLUE

| 1 | 2 | 3 | 4 | 5 |

Notes accompanying testicular pain

See also	Chart notes
Abdominal pain Unwell newborn	This is a presentation defined flow diagram. Testicular pain may have a number of pathologies, the most urgent of which is testicular torsion. A number of general discriminators are used including *Life threat*, *Pain* and *Temperature*. Specific discriminators included in the ORANGE category are designed to indicate those patients who have a high chance of torsion of the testes and the most severe infections. If the patient is under 28 days, the Unwell Newborn chart should be used

Specific discriminators	Explanation
Scrotal gangrene	Dead, blackened skin around the scrotum and groin. Early gangrene may not be black but may appear like a full-thickness burn with or without flaking
Age 25 years or less	A person aged less than 25 years
Scrotal cellulitis	Redness and swelling around the scrotum
Persistent vomiting	Vomiting that is continuous or that occurs without any respite between episodes
Colicky pain	Pain that comes and goes in waves. Renal colic tends to come and go over 20 minutes or so
Scrotal trauma	Any recent physically traumatic event involving the scrotum
Vomiting	Any emesis

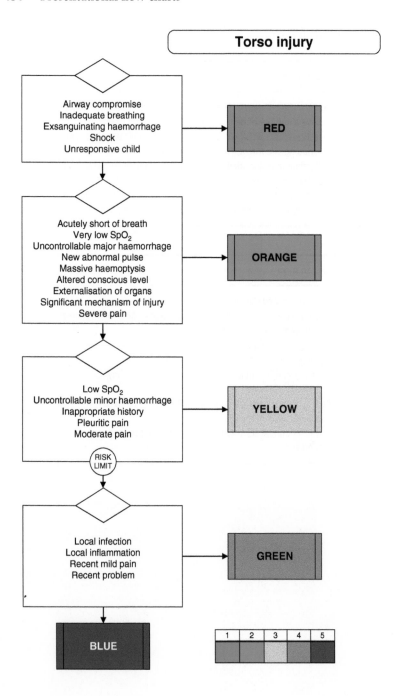

Torso injury

Airway compromise
Inadequate breathing
Exsanguinating haemorrhage
Shock
Unresponsive child

→ RED

Acutely short of breath
Very low SpO$_2$
Uncontrollable major haemorrhage
New abnormal pulse
Massive haemoptysis
Altered conscious level
Externalisation of organs
Significant mechanism of injury
Severe pain

→ ORANGE

Low SpO$_2$
Uncontrollable minor haemorrhage
Inappropriate history
Pleuritic pain
Moderate pain

→ YELLOW

RISK LIMIT

Local infection
Local inflammation
Recent mild pain
Recent problem

→ GREEN

BLUE

| 1 | 2 | 3 | 4 | 5 |

Notes accompanying torso injury

See also	Chart notes
Assault Major trauma Wounds	This is a presentation defined flow diagram designed to allow accurate prioritisation of patients who have suffered injuries to the front or back of the chest and abdomen. A number of general discriminators are used including *Life threat, Haemorrhage* and *Pain*. Specific discriminators have been used to allow the identification of patients who are suffering from less obvious but severe internal injury. These would include patients who are acutely short of breath and those with a history suggestive of significant trauma

Specific discriminators	Explanation
Acutely short of breath	Shortness of breath that comes on suddenly, or a sudden exacerbation of chronic shortness of breath
New abnormal pulse	A bradycardia (less than 60/minute in adults), a tachycardia (more than 100/minute in adults) or an irregular rhythm. Age appropriate definitions or bradycardia and tachycardia should be used in children
Very low SpO_2	This is a saturation of less than 95% on O_2 therapy or less than 92% on air
Low SpO_2	This is a saturation of less than 95% on air
Massive haemoptysis	Coughing up large amounts of fresh or clotted blood. Not to be confused with streaks of blood in saliva
Externalisation of organs	Herniation or frank extrusion of internal organs
Significant mechanism of injury	Penetrating injuries (stab or gunshot) and injuries with high energy transfer
Inappropriate history	When the history (story) given does not explain the physical findings it is termed inappropriate. This is important as it is a marker of safeguarding concerns in both adults and children
Pleuritic pain	A sharp, localised pain in the chest that worsens on breathing, coughing or sneezing
Local infection	Local infection usually manifests as inflammation (pain, swelling and redness) confined to a particular site or area, with or without a collection of pus
Local inflammation	Local inflammation will involve pain, swelling and redness confined to a particular site or area

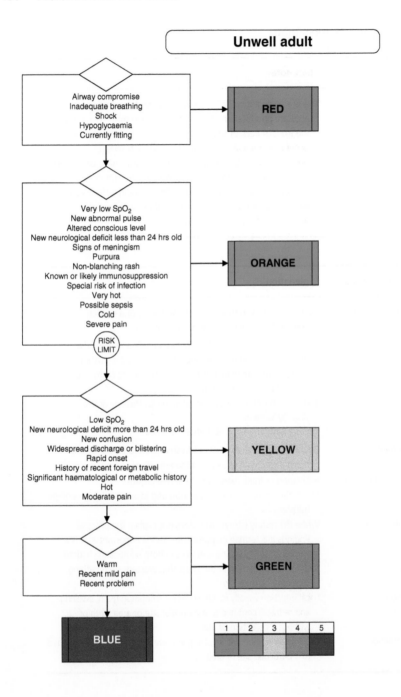

Notes accompanying unwell adult

See also	Chart notes
Collapse	This is a non-specific presentation defined flow diagram. A number of general discriminators are used including *Life threat*, *Conscious level*, *Pain* and *Temperature*. Specific discriminators have been included to ensure that patients with, for example, meningococcaemia are placed in the appropriate category

Specific discriminators	Explanation
Hypoglycaemia	Glucose less than 3 mmol/l
New abnormal pulse	A bradycardia (less than 60/min in adults), a tachycardia (more than 100/min in adults) or an irregular rhythm. Age-appropriate definitions of bradycardia and tachycardia should be used in children
Very low SpO_2	This is a saturation of less than 95% on O_2 therapy or less than 92% on air
New neurological deficit less than 24 hrs old	Any loss of neurological function that has come on within the previous 24 hours. This might include altered or lost sensation, weakness of the limbs (either transiently or permanently) and alterations in bladder or bowel function
Signs of meningism	Classically a stiff neck together with headache and photophobia
Purpura	A rash on any part of the body that is caused by small haemorrhages under the skin. A purpuric rash does not blanch (go white) when pressure is applied to it
Non-blanching rash	A rash that does not blanch (go white) when pressure is applied to it. Often tested using a glass tumbler to apply pressure as any colour change can be observed through the bottom of the tumbler
Known or likely immunosuppression	Any patient who is known to be immunosuppressed including those on immunosuppressive drugs (including long-term steroids)
Special risk of infection	Known exposure to a dangerous pathogen, or travel to an area with an identified, current, serious infectious risk
Possible sepsis	Suspected sepsis in patients who present with altered mental state, low blood pressure (systolic less than 100) or raised respiratory rate (rate more than 22). In children, age specific physiological tools should be used to determine if possibly septic
Low SpO_2	This is a saturation of less than 95% on air
New neurological deficit more than 24 hrs old	Any loss of neurological function including altered or lost sensation, weakness of the limbs (either transiently or permanently) and alterations in bladder or bowel function
New confusion	Patients with new onset confusion
Widespread discharge or blistering	Any discharging or blistering eruption covering more than 10% of the body surface area
Rapid onset	Onset within the preceding 12 hours
History of recent foreign travel	Recent significant foreign travel (within 2 weeks)
Significant haematological or metabolic history	A patient with significant haematological condition; or a congenital metabolic disorder that is known to deteriorate rapidly

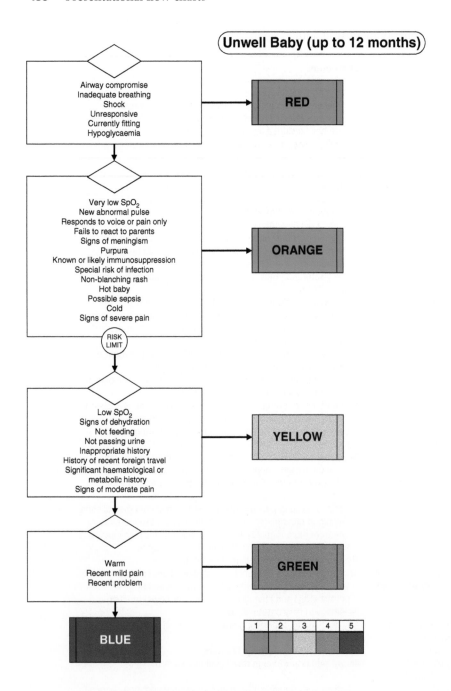

Unwell Baby (up to 12 months)

Airway compromise
Inadequate breathing
Shock
Unresponsive
Currently fitting
Hypoglycaemia

RED

Very low SpO$_2$
New abnormal pulse
Responds to voice or pain only
Fails to react to parents
Signs of meningism
Purpura
Known or likely immunosuppression
Special risk of infection
Non-blanching rash
Hot baby
Possible sepsis
Cold
Signs of severe pain

ORANGE

RISK LIMIT

Low SpO$_2$
Signs of dehydration
Not feeding
Not passing urine
Inappropriate history
History of recent foreign travel
Significant haematological or
metabolic history
Signs of moderate pain

YELLOW

Warm
Recent mild pain
Recent problem

GREEN

BLUE

| 1 | 2 | 3 | 4 | 5 |

Notes accompanying unwell baby (up to 12 months)

See also	Chart notes
Crying baby Unwell newborn Worried parent	This is a presentation defined flow diagram designed to allow accurate prioritisation of babies who present with non-specific illness. A number of general discriminators are used including *Life threat*, *Conscious level*, *Pain* and *Temperature*. A number of specific discriminators have been included to allow identification of more serious pathology such as meningococcaemia, etc. The risk limit sits between ORANGE and YELLOW and therefore no babies can be categorised as YELLOW, GREEN or BLUE until all the specific and general discriminators outlined under the RED and ORANGE categories have been specifically excluded. This may take longer than the time available for initial assessment. If the patient is under 28 days, the unwell newborn chart should be used

Specific discriminators	Explanation
Hypoglycaemia	Glucose less than 3 mmol/l
Very low SpO$_2$	This is a saturation of less than 95% on O$_2$ therapy or less than 92% on air
New abnormal pulse	Age-appropriate definitions of bradycardia and tachycardia should be used in children
Fails to react to parents	Failure to react in any way to a parent's face or voice. Abnormal reactions and apparent lack of recognition of a parent are also worrying signs
Signs of meningism	Classically a stiff neck together with headache and photophobia
Purpura	A rash on any part of the body that is caused by small haemorrhages under the skin. A purpuric rash does not blanch (go white) when pressure is applied to it
Known or likely immunosuppression	Any patient who is known or likely to be immunosuppressed including those on immunosuppressive drugs (including long-term steroids)
Special risk of infection	Known exposure to a dangerous pathogen, or travel to an area with an identified, current serious infectious risk
History of recent foreign travel	Recent significant foreign travel (within 2 weeks)
Non-blanching rash	A rash that does not blanch (go white) when pressure is applied to it. Often tested using a glass tumbler to apply pressure as any colour change can be observed through the bottom of the tumbler
Possible sepsis	Suspected sepsis in patients who present with altered mental state, low blood pressure (systolic less than 100) or raised respiratory rate (rate more than 22). In children, age specific physiological tools should be used to determine if possibly septic
Low SpO$_2$	This is a saturation of less than 95% on air
Signs of dehydration	These include dry tongue, sunken eyes, decreased skin turgor and, in small babies, a sunken anterior fontanelle. Usually associated with a low urine output
Not feeding	Children who will not take any solid or liquid (as appropriate) by mouth. Children who will take the food but always vomit afterwards may also fulfil this criterion
Not passing urine	Failure to produce and pass urine. This may be difficult to judge in children (and the elderly) and reference to the number of nappies or pads used may be useful
Inappropriate history	When the history (story) given does not explain the physical findings it is termed inappropriate. This is important as it is a marker of safeguarding concerns in both adults and children
Significant haematological or metabolic history	A patient with significant haematological condition; or a congenital metabolic disorder that is known to deteriorate rapidly

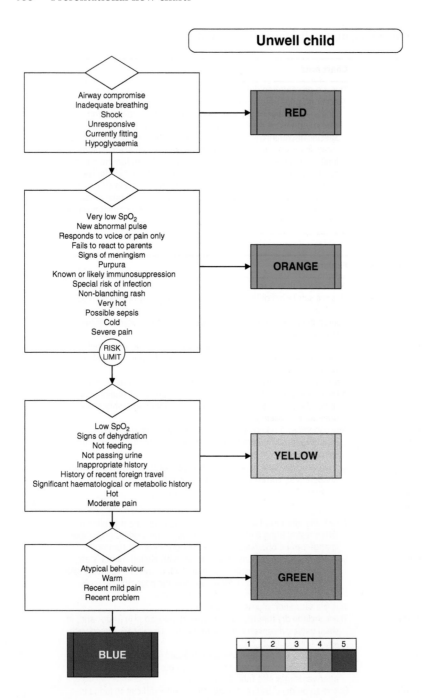

Notes accompanying unwell child

See also	Chart notes
Crying baby Irritable child Unwell newborn Worried parent	This is a presentation defined flow diagram designed to allow accurate prioritisation of children over the age of 12 months who present with non-specific illness. A number of general discriminators are used including *Life threat*, *Conscious level*, *Pain* and *Temperature*. A number of specific discriminators have been included to allow identification of more serious pathology such as meningococcaemia, etc. The risk limit sits between ORANGE and YELLOW and therefore no children can be categorised as YELLOW, GREEN or BLUE until all the specific and general discriminators outlined under the RED and ORANGE categories have been specifically excluded. This may take longer than the time available for initial assessment. If the patient is under 28 days, the Unwell Newborn chart should be used

Specific discriminators	Explanation
Hypoglycaemia	Glucose less than 3 mmol/l
Very low SpO_2	This is a saturation of less than 95% on O_2 therapy or less than 92% on air
New abnormal pulse	Age-appropriate definitions of bradycardia and tachycardia should be used in children
Fails to react to parents	Failure to react in any way to a parent's face or voice. Abnormal reactions and apparent lack of recognition of a parent are also worrying signs
Signs of meningism	Classically a stiff neck together with headache and photophobia
Purpura	A rash on any part of the body that is caused by small haemorrhages under the skin. A purpuric rash does not blanch (go white) when pressure is applied to it
Known or likely immunosuppression	Any patient who is known or likely to be immunosuppressed including those on immunosuppressive drugs (including long-term steroids)
Special risk of infection	Known exposure to a dangerous pathogen, or travel to an area with an an identified, current serious infectious risk
Non-blanching rash	A rash that does not blanch (go white) when pressure is applied to it. Often tested using a glass tumbler to apply pressure as any colour change can be observed through the bottom of the tumbler
Possible sepsis	Suspected sepsis in patients who present with altered mental state, low blood pressure (systolic less than 100) or raised respiratory rate (rate more than 22). In children, age specific physiological tools should be used to determine if possibly septic
Low SpO_2	This is a saturation of less than 95% on air
Signs of dehydration	These include dry tongue, sunken eyes, decreased skin turgor and, in small babies, a sunken anterior fontanelle. Usually associated with a low urine output
Not feeding	Children who will not take any solid or liquid (as appropriate) by mouth. Children who will take the food but always vomit afterwards may also fulfil this criterion
Not passing urine	Failure to produce and pass urine. This may be difficult to judge in children (and the elderly) and reference to the number of nappies or pads used may be useful
Inappropriate history	When the history (story) given does not explain the physical findings it is termed inappropriate. This is important as it is a marker of safeguarding concerns in both adults and children
History of recent foreign travel	Recent significant foreign travel (within 2 weeks)
Significant haematological or metabolic history	A patient with a significant haematological condition; or a congenital metabolic disorder that is known to deteriorate rapidly
Atypical behaviour	Children who are behaving in a way that is not usual in the given situation. The carers will often volunteer this information. Such children are often referred to as fractious or 'out of sorts'

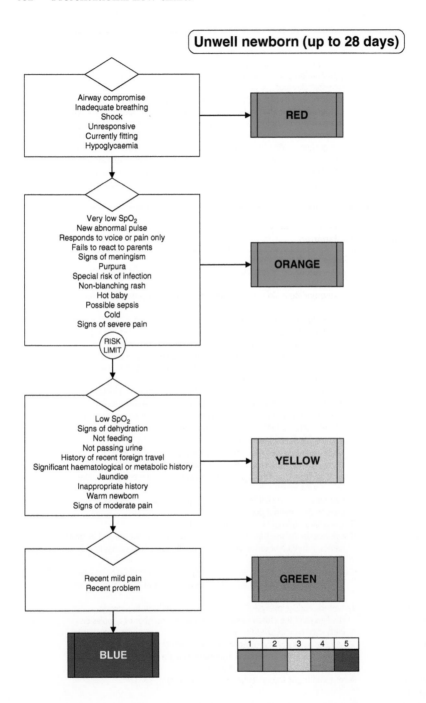

Unwell newborn (up to 28 days)

Airway compromise
Inadequate breathing
Shock
Unresponsive
Currently fitting
Hypoglycaemia

RED

Very low SpO$_2$
New abnormal pulse
Responds to voice or pain only
Fails to react to parents
Signs of meningism
Purpura
Special risk of infection
Non-blanching rash
Hot baby
Possible sepsis
Cold
Signs of severe pain

ORANGE

RISK LIMIT

Low SpO$_2$
Signs of dehydration
Not feeding
Not passing urine
History of recent foreign travel
Significant haematological or metabolic history
Jaundice
Inappropriate history
Warm newborn
Signs of moderate pain

YELLOW

Recent mild pain
Recent problem

GREEN

BLUE

1	2	3	4	5

Notes accompanying unwell newborn (up to 28 days)

See also	Chart notes
	This is a presentation defined flow diagram designed to allow accurate prioritisation of newborns (up to 28 days) who present with non-specific illness. A number of general discriminators are used including *Life threat*, *Conscious level*, *Pain* and *Temperature*. A number of specific discriminators have been included to allow identification of more serious pathology such as meningococcaemia, etc. The risk limit sits between ORANGE and YELLOW and therefore no newborns can be categorised as YELLOW, GREEN or BLUE until all the specific and general discriminators outlined under the RED and ORANGE categories have been specifically excluded. This may take longer than the time available for initial assessment

Specific discriminators	Explanation
Hypoglycaemia	Glucose less than 3 mmol/l
Very low SpO$_2$	This is a saturation of less than 95% on O$_2$ therapy or less than 92% on air
New abnormal pulse	Age-appropriate definitions of bradycardia and tachycardia should be used in children
Fails to react to parents	Failure to react in any way to a parent's face or voice. Abnormal reactions and apparent lack of recognition of a parent are also worrying signs
Signs of meningism	Classically a stiff neck together with headache and photophobia
Purpura	A rash on any part of the body that is caused by small haemorrhages under the skin. A purpuric rash does not blanch (go white) when pressure is applied to it
Special risk of infection	Known exposure to a dangerous pathogen, or travel to an area with an identified, current serious infectious risk
Non-blanching rash	A rash that does not blanch (go white) when pressure is applied to it. Often tested using a glass tumbler to apply pressure as any colour change can be observed through the bottom of the tumbler
Possible sepsis	Suspected sepsis in patients who present with altered mental state, low blood pressure (systolic less than 100) or raised respiratory rate (rate more than 22). In children, age specific physiological tools should be used to determine if possibly septic
Signs of severe pain	Young children and babies in severe pain cannot complain. They will usually cry out continuously and inconsolably and be tachycardic. They may well exhibit signs such as pallor and sweating
Low SpO$_2$	This is a saturation of less than 95% on air
Signs of dehydration	These include dry tongue, sunken eyes, decreased skin turgor and, in small babies, a sunken anterior fontanelle. Usually associated with a low urine output
Not feeding	Children who will not take any solid or liquid (as appropriate) by mouth. Children who will take the food but always vomit afterwards may also fulfil this criterion
Not passing urine	Failure to produce and pass urine. This may be difficult to judge in children (and the elderly) and reference to the number of nappies or pads used may be useful
History of recent foreign travel	Recent significant foreign travel (within 2 weeks)
Jaundice	Neonatal jaundice
Significant haematological or metabolic history	A patient with a significant haematological condition; or a congenital metabolic disorder that is known to deteriorate rapidly
Inappropriate history	When the history (story) given does not explain the physical findings it is termed inappropriate. This is important as it is a marker of safeguarding concerns in both adults and children
Signs of moderate pain	Young children and babies in moderate pain cannot complain. They will usually cry intermittently and are often intermittently consolable

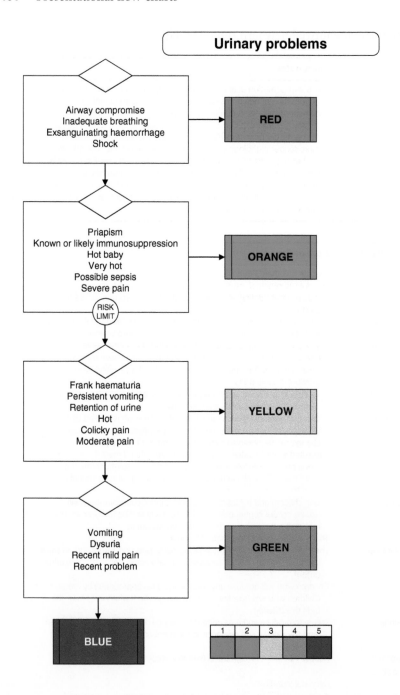

Notes accompanying urinary problems

See also	Chart notes
Sexually acquired infection Testicular pain Unwell newborn	This is a presentation defined flow diagram. A lot of patients who present with urinary problems are in pain and some may have serious underlying pathology. A number of general discriminators are used including *Life threat*, *Pain* and *Temperature*. Specific discriminators have been included to ensure that patients suffering from urinary retention and those with infections are included in the appropriate categories. If the patient is under 28 days, the Unwell newborn chart should be used

Specific discriminators	Explanation
Priapism	Sustained penile erection
Known or likely immunosuppression	Any patient who is known to be immunosuppressed including those on immunosuppressive drugs (including long-term steroids)
Possible sepsis	Suspected sepsis in patients who present with altered mental state, low blood pressure (systolic less than 100) or raised respiratory rate (rate more than 22). In children, age specific physiological tools should be used to determine if possibly septic
Frank haematuria	Red discolouration of the urine caused by blood
Persistent vomiting	Vomiting that is continuous or that occurs without any respite between episodes
Retention of urine	Inability to pass urine per urethra associated with an enlarged bladder. This condition is usually very painful unless there is altered sensation
Colicky pain	Pain that comes and goes in waves. Renal colic tends to come and go over 20 minutes or so
Dysuria	Pain or difficulty in passing urine. Pain is typically described as stinging or hot
Vomiting	Any emesis

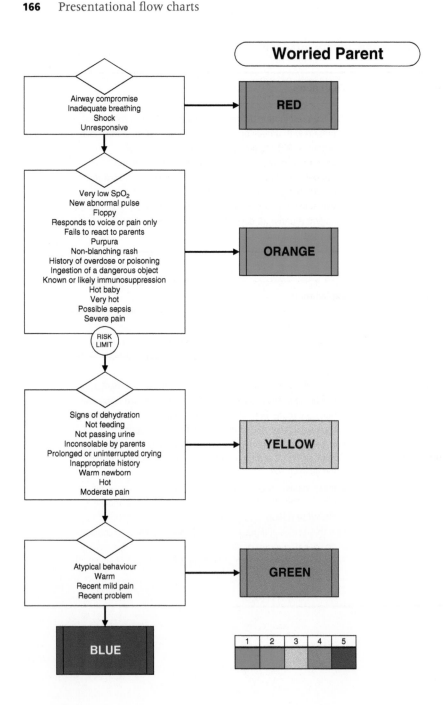

Notes accompanying worried parent

See also	Chart notes
Crying baby Irritable child Unwell baby Unwell child Unwell newborn	This is a presentation defined flow diagram that has been designed to allow accurate prioritisation of children who are brought to the attention of the service because of parental worry. Parents know their children better than anyone else and although many of these children will not have serious pathology it is essential that these presentations are taken seriously. A number of general discriminators are used including *Life threat*, *Conscious level*, *Pain* and *Temperature*. Specific discriminators have been added to the chart to allow identification of more serious pathologies which are apparent or may potentially exist. The risk limit sits between ORANGE and YELLOW and therefore no children can be categorised as YELLOW, GREEN or BLUE until all the specific and general discriminators outlined under the RED and ORANGE categories have been specifically excluded. This may take longer than the time available for initial assessment. If the patient is under 28 days, the Unwell Newborn chart should be used

Specific discriminators	Explanation
Very low SPO_2	This is a saturation of less the 95% O_2 theapy or less than 92% on air
Floppy	Parents may describe their children as floppy. Tone is generally reduced – the most noticeable sign is often lolling of the head
Fails to react to parents	Failure to react in any way to a parent's face or voice. Abnormal reactions and apparent lack of recognition of a parent are also worrying signs
Purpura	A rash on any part of the body that is caused by small haemorrhages under the skin. A purpuric rash does not blanch (go white) when pressure is applied to it
Non-blanching rash	A rash that does not blanch (go white) when pressure is applied to it. Often tested using a glass tumbler to apply pressure as any colour change can be observed through the bottom of the tumbler
History of overdose or poisoning	This information may come from others or may be deduced if medication is missing
Ingestion of a dangerous object	Ingestion of a dangerous or potentially dangerous foreign object e.g. button battery, magnets or razor blades which may be a potential threat to life
Known or likely immunosuppression	Any patient who is known to be immunosuppressed including those on immunosuppressive drugs (including long-term steroids)
Possible sepsis	Suspected sepsis in patients who present with altered mental state, low blood pressure (systolic less than 100) or raised respiratory rate (rate more than 22). In children, age specific physiological tools should be used to determine if possibly septic
Signs of dehydration	These include dry tongue, sunken eyes, decreased skin turgor and, in small babies, a sunken anterior fontanelle. Usually associated with a low urine output
Not feeding	Children who will not take any solid or liquid (as appropriate) by mouth. Children who will take the food but always vomit afterwards may also fulfil this criterion
Not passing urine	Failure to produce and pass urine. This may be difficult to judge in children (and the elderly) and reference to the number of nappies or pads used may be useful
Inconsolable by parents	Children whose crying or distress does not respond to attempts by their parents to comfort them
Prolonged or uninterrupted crying	A child who has cried continuously for 2 hours or more
Inappropriate history	When the history (story) given does not explain the physical findings it is termed inappropriate. This is important as it is a marker of safeguarding concerns in both adults and children
Atypical behaviour	Children who are behaving in a way that is not usual in the given situation. The carers will often volunteer this information. Such children are often referred to as fractious or 'out of sorts'

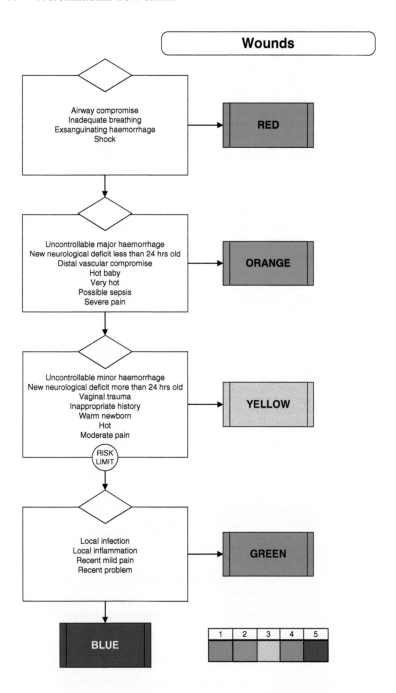

Wounds

Airway compromise
Inadequate breathing
Exsanguinating haemorrhage
Shock

RED

Uncontrollable major haemorrhage
New neurological deficit less than 24 hrs old
Distal vascular compromise
Hot baby
Very hot
Possible sepsis
Severe pain

ORANGE

Uncontrollable minor haemorrhage
New neurological deficit more than 24 hrs old
Vaginal trauma
Inappropriate history
Warm newborn
Hot
Moderate pain

RISK LIMIT

YELLOW

Local infection
Local inflammation
Recent mild pain
Recent problem

GREEN

BLUE

Notes accompanying wounds

See also	Chart notes
Assault	This is a presentation defined flow diagram. Many patients attend all forms of emergency care suffering from wounds of varying nature. These vary from severe life-threatening lacerations to minor abrasions. This chart is designed to allow an accurate prioritisation of these patients. A number of general discriminators have been used including *Life threat*, *Haemorrhage* and *Pain*. Specific discriminators have been included to allow identification of patients with signs and symptoms suggesting injuries that pose a threat to function

Specific discriminators	Explanation
Distal vascular compromise	There will be a combination of pallor, coldness, altered sensation and pain with or without absent pulses distal to the injury
Possible sepsis	Suspected sepsis in patients who present with altered mental state, low blood pressure (systolic less than 100) or raised respiratory rate (rate more than 22). In children, age specific physiological tools should be used to determine if possibly septic
New neurological deficit more than 24 hrs old	Any loss of neurological function including altered or lost sensation, weakness of the limbs (either transiently or permanently) and alterations in bladder or bowel function
Vaginal trauma	Any history or other evidence of direct trauma to the vagina
Inappropriate history	When the history (story) given does not explain the physical findings it is termed inappropriate. This is important as it is a marker of safeguarding concerns in both adults and children
Local infection	Local infection usually manifests as inflammation (pain, swelling and redness) confined to a particular site or area, with or without a collection of pus
Local inflammation	Local inflammation will involve pain, swelling and redness confined to a particular site or area

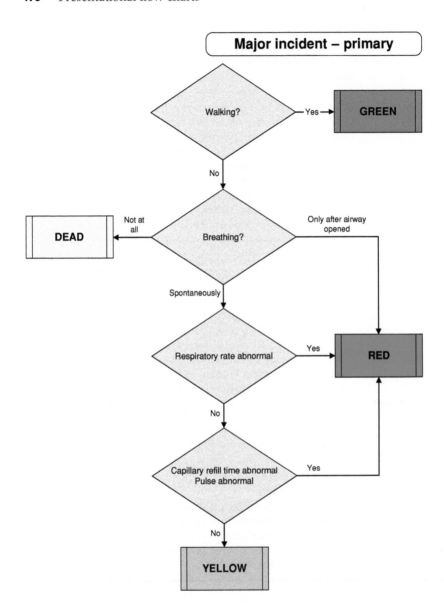

Notes accompanying major incident – primary

See also	Chart notes
Major incidents – secondary	Triage during a major incident has a completely different aim from that during the day-to-day running of emergency services. To achieve this aim (which is to initially save as many lives as possible and then to deliver the best care possible within the existing resources) a different approach has been taken. Rather than select the most seriously ill first, in this instance the least ill are selected. Rather than using general and specific discriminators, very broad brush discriminators are used that allow rough division of patients into three categories. This chart describes the first 'sorting' triage method for use in major incidents. It is designed to allow rapid imposition of order when a large number of untriaged casualties arrive at once. It does not pick out the most severe first, rather selecting the most numerous (walking) and then subcategorising the stretcher patients as dead, red or yellow. Inevitably this quick method is not totally accurate, and other methods should be used once time allows. No longer than 15 seconds should be spent on each patient

Specific discriminators	Explanation
Walking	The ability to walk (whatever the injury) is used as a discriminator to select patients of the standard category
Breathing after airway opened	Patients who cannot breathe after their airway is opened are considered dead unless considerable life support resources exist
Respiratory rate abnormal	Casualties whose respiratory rate is abnormal either by being too high (over 29 breaths/min) or too low (less than 10 breaths/min) are categorised as RED
Capillary refill time abnormal	Casualties whose capillary refill is prolonged (more than 2 seconds) are categorised as RED
Pulse abnormal	If the capillary refill time cannot be measured then casualties whose pulse is raised over 120/min are categorised as RED
	All other patients are placed in the YELLOW category

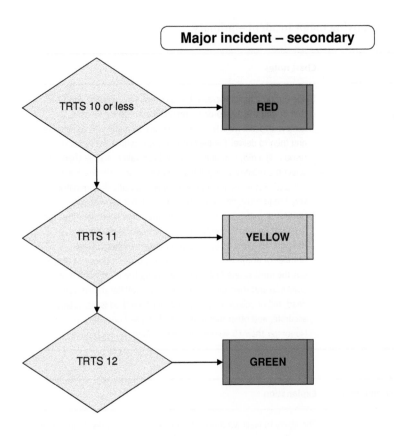

Notes accompanying major incident – secondary

See also	Chart notes
Major incidents – primary	The primary major incident triage methodology is used to rapidly screen a large number of patients into broad brush categories. The Triage Revised Trauma Score (TRTS) is a slightly more refined physiological approach to the triage of a large number of casualties. It is based on the coded values of three physiological parameters. Priorities are allocated from the TRTS as follows:
	1–10: Priority 1 (RED)
	11: Priority 2 (YELLOW)
	12: Priority 3 (GREEN)
	(0: Priority 4)

Specific discriminators	Explanation
TRTS	Triage Revised Trauma Score
Respiratory rate (breaths/min)	
10–29	4
>29	3
6–9	2
1–5	1
0	0
Systolic blood pressure (mmHg)	
90	4
76–89	3
50–75	2
1–49	1
0	0
Glasgow Coma Scale score	
13–15	4
9–12	3
6–8	2
4–5	1
3	0

Discriminator dictionary

Abdominal pain	Any pain felt in the abdomen. Abdominal pain associated with back pain may indicate abdominal aortic aneurysm, while association with PV bleeding may indicate ectopic pregnancy or miscarriage
Abrupt onset	Onset within seconds or minutes. May cause waking from sleep
Acute chemical eye injury	Any substance splashed into or placed into the eye within the past 12 hours that caused stinging, burning or reduced vision should be assumed to have caused chemical injury
Acute complete loss of vision	Loss of vision in one or both eyes within the preceding 24 hours that has not returned to normal
Acute onset after injury	Onset of symptoms immediately within 24 hours of a physically traumatic event
Acutely avulsed tooth	A tooth that has been avulsed intact within the previous 24 hours
Acutely short of breath	Shortness of breath that comes on suddenly, or a sudden exacerbation of chronic shortness of breath
Age 25 years or less	A person aged less than 25 years
Airway compromise	An airway may be compromised either because it cannot be kept open or because the airway protective reflexes (that stop inhalation) have been lost. Failure to keep the airway open will result either in intermittent total obstruction or in partial obstruction. This will manifest itself as snoring or bubbling sounds during breathing
Altered conscious level	Not fully alert. Either responding to voice or pain only or unresponsive
Altered conscious level *not* wholly attributable to alcohol	A patient who is not fully alert, with a history of alcohol ingestion, and in whom there may be other causes of reduced conscious level

---

Emergency Triage: Manchester Triage Group, Third Edition.
Edited by Kevin Mackway-Jones, Janet Marsden and Jill Windle.
© 2014 John Wiley & Sons, Ltd. Published 2014 by John Wiley & Sons, Ltd.

Altered conscious level wholly attributable to alcohol	A patient who is not fully alert, with a clear history of alcohol ingestion and in whom there is no doubt that all other causes of reduced conscious level have been excluded
Altered facial sensation	Any alteration of sensation on the face
Aortic pain	The onset of symptoms is sudden and the leading symptom is severe abdominal or chest pain. The pain may be described as sharp, stabbing or ripping in character. Classically aortic chest pain is felt around the sternum and then radiates to the shoulder blades, aortic abdominal pain is felt in the centre of the abdomen and radiates to the back. The pain may get better or even vanish and then recur elsewhere. Over time, pain may also be felt in the arms, neck, lower jaw, stomach or hips.
Apparently hallucinating	Patients who are apparently hallucinating may appear distracted and may appear to react to stimuli (primarily visual and auditory) that are not apparent to anyone else
Atypical behaviour	Children who are behaving in a way that is not usual in the given situation. The carers will often volunteer this information. Such children are often referred to as fractious or 'out of sorts'
Auricular haematoma	A tense haematoma (usually post traumatic) in the outer ear
Black or redcurrant stool	Any blackness fulfils the criteria of black stool while a dark red stool, classically seen in intussusceptions, is redcurrant stool
Bleeding disorder	Congenital or acquired bleeding disorder
Cardiac pain	Classically a severe, dull, 'gripping' or 'heavy' pain in the centre of the chest, radiating to the left arm or to the neck. May be associated with sweating and nausea
Chest injury	Any injury to the area below the clavicles and above the level of the lowest rib. Injury to the lower part of the chest can cause underlying damage to abdominal organs
Cold	If the skin feels cold the patient is clinically said to be cold. The temperature should be taken as soon as possible - a core temperature less than 35°C is cold
Colicky pain	Pain that comes and goes in waves. Renal colic tends to come and go over 20 minutes or so

Critical skin	A fracture or dislocation may leave fragments or ends of bone pressing so hard against the skin that the viability of the skin is threatened. The skin will be white and under tension
Current palpitation	A feeling of the heart racing (often described as a fluttering) that is still present
Currently fitting	Patients who are in the tonic or clonic stages of a grand mal convulsion, and patients currently experiencing partial fits
Deformity	This will always be subjective. Abnormal angulation or rotation is implied
Diplopia	Double vision that resolves when one eye is closed
Direct trauma to the back	This may be top to bottom (loading), for instance when people fall and land on their feet, bending (forwards, backwards or to the side) or twisting
Direct trauma to the neck	This may be top to bottom (loading), for instance when something falls on the head, bending (forwards, backwards or to the side), twisting or distracting such as in hanging
Discharge	In the context of sexually acquired infection this is any discharge from the penis or abnormal discharge from the vagina
Discharged from mental health services within the past 15 days	Any patient who has been discharged from an active period of care under mental health services (in hospital or in the community) within the past 15 days
Disruptive	Disruptive behaviour is behaviour that affects the smooth running of the department. It may be threatening
Distal vascular compromise	There will be a combination of pallor, coldness, altered sensation and pain with or without absent pulses distal to the injury
Drooling	Saliva running from the mouth as a result of being unable to swallow
Dysuria	Pain or difficulty in passing urine. Pain is typically described as stinging or hot
Electrical injury	Any injury caused or possibly caused by an electric current. This includes AC and DC and both artificial and natural sources
Exhaustion	Exhausted patients appear to reduce the effort they make to breathe despite continuing respiratory insufficiency. This is pre-terminal
Exsanguinating haemorrhage	Haemorrhage which is occurring at such a rate that death will ensue unless bleeding is stopped
Externalisation of organs	Herniation or frank extrusion of internal organs

Extreme aggression or agitation requiring immediate restraint	Aggression and agitation of such a degree that immediate restraint is required to manage the risk of harm to self or others
Facial oedema	Diffuse swelling around the face, usually involving the lips
Facial swelling	Swelling around the face which may be localised or diffuse
Fails to react to parents	Failure to react in any way to a parent's face or voice. Abnormal reactions and apparent lack of recognition of a parent are also worrying signs
Floppy	Parents may describe their children as floppy. Tone is generally reduced - the most noticeable sign is often lolling of the head
Foreign body sensation	A sensation of something in the eye, often expressed as scraping or grittiness
Frank haematuria	Red discolouration of the urine caused by blood
Gross deformity	This will always be subjective. Gross and abnormal angulation or rotation is implied
Headache	Any pain around the head that is not related to a particular anatomical structure. Facial pain is not included
Heavy PV blood loss	PV loss is extremely difficult to assess. The presence of large clots or constant flow fulfils this criterion. The use of a large number of sanitary towels is suggestive of heavy loss
High blood pressure	A history of raised blood pressure or a raised blood pressure on examination
High lethality	Lethality is the potential of the substance taken to cause harm. Advice from a poisons centre may be required to establish the level of risk of serious illness or death. If in doubt, assume a high risk
High lethality chemical	Lethality is the potential of the chemical to cause harm. Advice may be required to establish the level of risk. If in doubt, assume a high risk
High lethality envenomation	Lethality is the potential of the envenomation to cause harm. Local knowledge may allow identification of the venomous creature, but advice may be required. If in doubt, assume a high risk
High risk of further self harm	An initial view of the risk of harm to self can be formed by considering the patient's behaviour. Patients who are threatening to harm themselves and who are actively seeking the means to do so are at high risk
High risk of leaving before assessment	Active, credible threats to leave prior to assessment pose a high risk
High risk of self harm	An initial view of the risk of harm to self can be formed by considering the patient's behaviour. Patients who are threatening to harm themselves and who are actively seeking the means to do so are at high risk

History of acutely vomiting blood	Frank haematemesis, vomiting of altered blood (coffee ground) or of blood mixed in the vomit within the past 24 hours
History of fitting	Any observed or reported fits that have occurred during the period of illness or following an episode of trauma
History of head injury	A history of a recent physically traumatic event involving the head. Usually this will be reported by the patient but if the patient has been unconscious this history should be sought from a reliable witness
History of overdose or poisoning	This information may come from others or may be deduced if medication is missing
History of recent foreign travel	Recent significant foreign travel (within 2 weeks)
History of trauma	A history of a recent physically traumatic event
History of unconsciousness	There may be a reliable witness who can state whether the patient was unconscious (and for how long). If not, a patient who is unable to remember the incident should be assumed to have been unconscious
Hot	If the skin feels hot the person is clinically said to be hot. The temperature should be taken as soon as possible - a temperature of 38.5°C and greater is hot
Hot baby	If the skin is hot, the child is clinically said to be hot. The temperature should be taken as soon as possible - a temperature of 38.5°C and greater is hot. A baby is a child less than 1 year old
Hot joint	Any warmth around a joint. Often accompanied by redness
Hyperglycaemia	Glucose greater than 17 mmol/l
Hyperglycaemia with ketosis	Glucose greater than 11 mmol/l with urinary ketones or signs of acidosis (deep sighing respiration, etc.)
Hypoglycaemia	Glucose less than 3 mmol/l
Immediate risk of leaving before assessment	Active, credible attempts to leave prior to assessment pose an immediate risk
Immediate risk to others	An initial view of the risk of harm to others can be judged by looking at posture (tense, clenched), speech (loud, using threatening words) and motor behaviour (restless, pacing, lunging at others). Immediate risk should be assumed if weapons and potential victims are available and no controls are already in place.
Immediate risk to self	An initial view of the risk of harm to self can be formed by considering the patient's behaviour. Patients who are actively harming themselves and those who are threatening to harm themselves and who have the means to do so are at immediate risk
In active labour	A woman who is having regular and frequent painful contractions

Inadequate breathing	Patients who are failing to breathe well enough to maintain adequate oxygenation have inadequate breathing. There may be an increased work of breathing, signs of inadequate breathing or exhaustion
Inadequate history	If there is no clear and unequivocal history of acute alcohol ingestion, and if head injury, drug ingestion, underlying medical condition, etc. cannot be definitely excluded, then the history is inadequate
Inappropriate history	When the history (story) given does not explain the physical findings it is termed inappropriate. This is important as it is a marker of safeguarding concerns in both adults and children
Inconsolable by parents	Children whose crying or distress does not respond to attempts by their parents to comfort them
Increased work of breathing	Increased work of breathing is shown as increased respiratory rate, use of accessory muscles and grunting
Ingestion of a dangerous object	Ingestion of a dangerous or potentially dangerous foreign object e.g. button battery, magnets or razor blades which may be a potential threat to life
Inhalational injury	A history of being confined in a smoke-filled space is the most reliable indicator of smoke inhalation. Carbon deposits around the mouth and nose and hoarse voice may be present. History is also the most reliable way of diagnosing inhalation of chemicals - there will not necessarily be any signs
Jaundice	Neonatal jaundice
Known or likely immunosuppression	Any patient who is known or likely to be immunosuppressed including those on immunosuppressive drugs (including long-term steroids)
Likely to require admission under mental health legislation	Patients with significant psychiatric symptoms who are likely to require admission under mental health legislation
Local infection	Local infection usually manifests as inflammation (pain, swelling and redness) confined to a particular site or area, with or without a collection of pus
Local inflammation	Local inflammation will involve pain, swelling and redness confined to a particular site or area
Low PEFR	The PEFR predicted after consideration of the age and sex of the patient. Some patients may know their 'best' PEFR and this may be used. If the ratio of measured to predicted is less than 50% then this criterion is fulfilled
Low SpO_2	This is a saturation of less than 95% on air
Lower abdominal pain	Any pain felt in the lower abdomen; association with PV bleeding may indicate ectopic pregnancy or miscarriage

Marked distress	Patients who are markedly physically or emotionally upset
Massive haemoptysis	Coughing up large amounts of fresh or clotted blood. Not to be confused with streaks of blood in saliva
Moderate aggression or agitation	Agitation or aggression that can usually be managed by verbal de-escalation without physical restraint
Moderate itch	An itch that is bearable but intense
Moderate lethality	Lethality is the potential of the substance taken to cause serious illness or death. Advice from a poisons centre may be required to establish the level of risk to the patient
Moderate lethality chemical	Lethality is the potential of the chemical to cause harm. Advice may be required to establish the level of risk. If in doubt, assume a high risk
Moderate lethality envenomation	Lethality is the potential of the envenomation to cause harm. Local knowledge may allow identification of the venomous creature, but advice may be required
Moderate pain	Pain that is bearable but intense
Moderate risk of further self harm	An initial view of the risk of harm to self can be formed by considering the patient's behaviour. Patients without a significant history of self harm, who are not actively trying to harm themselves, but who profess the desire to harm themselves are at moderate risk
Moderate risk of harm to others	An initial view of the risk of harm to others can be judged by looking at posture (tense, clenched), speech (loud, using threatening words) and motor behaviour (restless, pacing, lunging at others). Moderate risk should be assumed if there is any indication of potential harm to others
Moderate risk of leaving before assessment	Threats to leave without any attempts to do so pose a moderate risk
Moderate risk of self harm	An initial view of the risk of harm to self can be formed by considering the patient's behaviour. Patients without a significant history of self harm, who are not actively trying to harm themselves, but who profess the desire to harm themselves are at moderate risk
New abnormal pulse	A bradycardia (less than 60/min in adults), a tachycardia (more than 100/min in adults) or an irregular rhythm. Age-appropriate definitions of bradycardia and tachycardia should be used in children
New confusion	Patients with new onset confusion
New neurological deficit less than 24 hours old	Any loss of neurological function that has come on within the previous 24 hours. This might include altered or lost sensation, weakness of the limbs (either transiently or permanently) and alterations in bladder or bowel function

New neurological deficit more than 24 hours old — Any loss of neurological function including altered or lost sensation, weakness of the limbs (either transiently or permanently) and alterations in bladder or bowel function

New onset of significant mental health symptoms — Any new mental health symptoms not already taken into account

New symptoms of psychosis — Active new symptoms of psychosis with no insight such as hallucinations, delusions and/or paranoia

No improvement with own asthma medications — This history should be available from the patient. A failure to improve with bronchodilator therapy given by the GP or paramedic is equally significant

Non-blanching rash — A rash that does not blanch (go white) when pressure is applied to it. Often tested using a glass tumbler to apply pressure as any colour change can be observed through the bottom of the tumbler

Not distractible — Children who are distressed by pain or other things who cannot be distracted by conversation or play

Not feeding — Children who will not take any solid or liquid (as appropriate) by mouth. Children who will take the food but always vomit afterwards may also fulfil this criterion

Not passing urine — Failure to produce and pass urine. This may be difficult to judge in children (and the elderly) and reference to the number of nappies or pads used may be useful

Oedema of the tongue — Swelling of the tongue of any degree

Open fracture — All wounds in the vicinity of a fracture should be regarded with suspicion. If there is any possibility of communication between the wound and the fracture then the fracture should be assumed to be open

Pain on joint movement — This can be pain on either active (patient) movement or passive (examiner) movement

Passing fresh or altered blood PR — In active massive GI bleeding, dark red blood will be passed PR. As GI transit time increases this becomes darker, eventually becoming melaena

Penetrating eye injury — A recent physically traumatic event involving penetration of the globe

Persistent vomiting — Vomiting that is continuous or that occurs without any respite between episodes

Pleuritic pain — A sharp, localised pain in the chest that worsens on breathing, coughing or sneezing

Possible sepsis — Suspected sepsis in patients who present with altered mental state, low blood pressure (Systolic less than 100) or raised respiratory rate (rate more than 22). In children, age specific physiological tools should be used to determine if possibly septic

Possibly pregnant — Any woman whose normal menstruation has failed to occur is possibly pregnant. Furthermore any woman of childbearing age who is having unprotected sex should be considered to be potentially pregnant

Presenting foetal parts	Crowning or presentation of any other foetal part in the vagina
Priapism	Sustained penile erection
Productive cough	A cough that is productive of phlegm, whatever the colour
Prolapsed umbilical cord	Prolapse of any part of the umbilical cord through the cervix
Prolonged or uninterrupted crying	A child who has cried continuously for 2 hours or more
Purpura	A rash on any part of the body that is caused by small haemorrhages under the skin. A purpuric rash does not blanch (go white) when pressure is applied to it
PV blood loss	Any loss of blood PV
PV blood loss and 20 weeks pregnant or more	Any loss of blood PV in a woman known to be beyond the 20th week of pregnancy
Rapid onset	Onset within the preceding 12 hours
Recent hearing loss	Loss of hearing in one or both ears within the previous week
Recent injury	An injury occurring within the last week
Recent mild itch	Any itch that has occurred in the past 7 days
Recent mild pain	Any pain that has occurred within the past 7 days
Recent problem	A problem arising in the last week
Recent reduced visual acuity	Any reduction in corrected visual acuity within the past 7 days
Recent signs of mild pain	Young children and babies in pain cannot complain. They will usually cry occasionally and may act atypically
Recently given birth	A woman who has given birth within the past 3 months
Red eye	Any redness to the eye. A red eye may be painful or painless and may be complete or partial
Reduced foetal movements >20 weeks	Absent or reduced foetal movements during the previous 12 hours in a woman known to be beyond the 20th week of pregnancy
Responds to pain	Response to a painful stimulus. Standard peripheral stimuli should be used - a pencil or pen is used to apply pressure to the finger nail bed. This stimulus should not be applied to the toes since a spinal reflex may cause flexion even in brain death. Supraorbital ridge pressure should not be used since reflex grimacing may occur
Responds to voice	Response to a vocal stimulus. It is not necessary to shout the patient's name. Children may fail to respond because they are afraid

Responds to voice or pain only	Responds to a vocal or painful stimulus
Retention of urine	Inability to pass urine per urethra associated with an enlarged bladder. This condition is usually very painful unless there is altered sensation
Risk of continued contamination	If chemical exposure is likely to continue (usually due to lack of adequate decontamination) then this discriminator applies. Risks to health care workers must not be forgotten if this situation occurs
Safeguarding concerns	Any concerns for the welfare of the patient that arise from their vulnerability
Scalp haematoma	A raised bruised area to the scalp (bruises below the hair line at the front are to the forehead)
Scrotal cellulitis	Redness and swelling around the scrotum
Scrotal gangrene	Dead, blackened skin around the scrotum and groin. Early gangrene may not be black but may appear like a full-thickness burn with or without flaking
Scrotal trauma	Any recent physically traumatic event involving the scrotum
Self harmed without other psychiatric disease	Patients who have harmed themselves (for the first or subsequent time) who do not have a mental health diagnosis
Severe aggression or agitation that may require restraint	Aggression and agitation of such a degree that restraint may be required at short notice to manage the risk of harm to self or others
Severe itch	An itch that is unbearable
Severe pain	Pain that is unbearable - often described as the worst ever
Shock	Shock is inadequate delivery of oxygen to the tissues. The classic signs include sweating, pallor, tachycardia, hypotension and reduced conscious level
Shoulder tip pain	Pain felt in the tip of the shoulder. This often indicates diaphragmatic irritation
Significant cardiac history	A known recurrent dysrhythmia that has life-threatening effects is significant, as is a known cardiac condition which may deteriorate rapidly
Significant haematological or metabolic history	A patient with a significant haematological condition or a congenital metabolic disorder that is known to deteriorate rapidly
Significant history of allergy	A known sensitivity with severe reaction (e.g. to nuts or bee sting) is significant
Significant history of GI bleed	Any history of massive GI bleeding or of any GI bleed associated with oesophageal varices
Significant mechanism of injury	Penetrating injuries (stab or gunshot) and injuries with high energy transfer
Significant medical history	Any preexisting medical condition requiring continual medication or other care

Significant psychiatric history	A history of a major psychiatric illness or event
Significant respiratory history	A history of previous life-threatening episodes of a respiratory condition (e.g. COPD) is significant, as is brittle asthma
Signs of dehydration	These include dry tongue, sunken eyes, decreased skin turgor and, in small babies, a sunken anterior fontanelle. Usually associated with a low urine output
Signs of meningism	Classically a stiff neck together with headache and photophobia
Signs of moderate pain	Young children and babies in moderate pain cannot complain. They will usually cry intermittently and are often intermittently consolable
Signs of severe pain	Young children and babies in severe pain cannot complain. They will usually cry out continuously and inconsolably and be tachycardic. They may well exhibit signs such as pallor and sweating
Smoke exposure	Smoke inhalation should be assumed if the patient has been confined in a smoke-filled space. Physical signs such as oral or nasal soot are less reliable but significant if present
Special risk of infection	Known exposure to a dangerous pathogen, or travel to an area with an identified, current serious infectious risk
Stridor	This may be an inspiratory or expiratory noise, or both. Stridor is heard best on breathing with the mouth open
Subcutaneous gas	Gas under the skin can be detected by feeling for a 'crackling' on touch. There may be gas bubbles and a line of demarcation
Swelling	An abnormal increase in size
Temporal scalp tenderness	Tenderness on palpation over the temporal area (especially over the artery)
Testicular pain	Pain in the testicles
Threats of violence or high risk of harm to others	An initial view of the risk of harm to others can be judged by looking at posture (tense, clenched), speech (loud, using threatening words) and motor behaviour (restless, pacing, lunging at others). High risk should be assumed if potential victims are available and inadequate controls are in place
Unable to feed	This is usually reported by the parents. Children who will not take any solid or liquid (as appropriate) by mouth
Unable to talk in sentences	Patients who are so breathless that they cannot complete relatively short sentences in one breath

Unable to walk	It is important to try and distinguish between patients who have pain and difficulty walking and those who *cannot* walk. Only the latter can be said to be unable to walk
Uncontrollable major haemorrhage	A haemorrhage that is not rapidly controlled by the application of sustained direct pressure and in which blood continues to flow heavily or soak through large dressings quickly
Uncontrollable minor haemorrhage	A haemorrhage that is not rapidly controlled by the application of sustained direct pressure and in which blood continues to flow slightly or ooze
Unresponsive	Patients who fail to respond to either verbal or painful stimuli
Unresponsive child	A child who fails to respond to either verbal or painful stimuli
Vaginal trauma	Any history or other evidence of direct trauma to the vagina
Vascular compromise	There will be a combination of pallor, coldness, altered sensation and pain with or without absent pulses distal to the injury
Vertigo	An acute feeling of spinning or dizziness, possibly accompanied by nausea and vomiting
Very hot	If the skin feels very hot the patient is clinically said to be very hot. The temperature should be taken as soon as possible - a temperature of 41°C or greater is very hot
Very low PEFR	The PEFR predicted after consideration of the age and sex of the patient. Some patients may know their 'best' PEFR and this may be used. If the ratio of measured to predicted is less than 33% then this criterion is fulfilled
Very low SpO_2	This is a saturation of less than 95% on O_2 therapy or less than 92% on air
Visible abdominal mass	A mass in the abdomen that is visible to the naked eye
Vomiting	Any emesis
Vomiting blood	Vomited blood may be fresh (bright or dark red) or coffee ground in appearance
Warm	If the skin feels warm the patient is clinically said to be warm. The temperature should be taken as soon as possible - a temperature greater than 37.5°C is warm
Warm newborn	If the skin feels warm the patient is clinically said to be warm. The temperature should be taken as soon as possible - a child of 28 days or under with a temperature of 37.5-38.4°C is warm

Wheeze	This can be audible wheeze or a feeling of wheeze. Very severe airway obstruction is silent (no air can move)
Widespread discharge or blistering	Any discharging or blistering eruption covering more than 10% of the body surface area
Widespread rash or blistering	Any rash or blistering eruption covering more than 10% of the body surface area

Index

Page references for the presentational flow charts and chart notes are given in bold type, e.g. chest pain **90–1**.

Emergency Triage: Manchester Triage Group, Third Edition.
Edited by Kevin Mackway-Jones, Janet Marsden and Jill Windle.
© 2014 John Wiley & Sons, Ltd. Published 2014 by John Wiley & Sons, Ltd.

General discriminator	Explanation
Airway compromise	An airway may be compromised either because it cannot be kept open or because the airway protective reflexes (that stop inhalation) have been lost. Failure to keep the airway open will result either in intermittent total obstruction or in partial obstruction. This will manifest itself as snoring or bubbling sounds during breathing
Inadequate breathing	Patients who are failing to breathe well enough to maintain adequate oxygenation have inadequate breathing. There may be an increased work of breathing, signs of inadequate breathing or exhaustion
Exsanguinating haemorrhage	Haemorrhage which is occurring at such a rate that death will ensue unless bleeding is stopped
Shock	Shock is inadequate delivery of oxygen to the tissues. The classic signs include sweating, pallor, tachycardia, hypotension and reduced conscious level
Unresponsive child	A child who fails to respond to either verbal or painful stimuli
Currently fitting	Patients who are in the tonic or clonic stages of a grand mal convulsion, and patients currently experiencing partial fits
Altered conscious level	Not fully alert. Either responding to voice or pain or unresponsive
Responds to pain	Response to a painful stimulus. Standard peripheral stimuli should be used – a pencil or pen is used to apply pressure to the finger nail bed. This stimulus should not be applied to the toes since a spinal reflex may cause flexion even in brain death. Supraorbital ridge pressure should not be used since reflex grimacing may occur
Responds to voice	Response to a vocal stimulus. It is not necessary to shout the patient's name. Children may fail to respond because they are afraid
Uncontrollable major haemorrhage	A haemorrhage that is not rapidly controlled by the application of a sustained direct pressure and in which blood continues to flow heavily or soak through large dressings quickly
Very hot	If the skin feels very hot the patient is clinically said to be very hot. The temperature should be taken as soon as possible – a temperature of 41°C or greater is very hot
Hot baby	If the skin is hot, the child is clinically said to be hot. The temperature should be taken as soon as possible – a temperature of 38.5°C and greater is hot. A baby is a child less than 1 year old
Cold	If the skin feels cold the patient is clinically said to be cold. The temperature should be taken as soon as possible – a core temperature less than 35°C is cold
Severe pain	Pain that is unbearable – often described as the worst ever (see chapter 4)
Uncontrollable minor haemorrhage	A haemorrhage that is not rapidly controlled by the application of sustained direct pressure and in which blood continues to flow slightly or ooze
History of unconsciousness	There may be a reliable witness who can state whether the patient was unconscious (and for how long). If not, a patient who is unable to remember the incident should be assumed to have been unconscious
Warm newborn	If the skin feels warm the patient is clinically said to be warm. The temperature should be taken as soon as possible – a child of 28 days or under with a temperature of 37.5–38.4°C is warm
Hot	If the skin feels hot the person is clinically said to be hot. The temperature should be taken as soon as possible – a temperature of 38.5°C and greater is hot
Moderate pain	Pain that is bearable but intense (see chapter 4)
Warm	If the skin feels warm the patient is clinically said to be warm. The temperature should be taken as soon as possible – a temperature greater than 37.5°C is warm
Recent mild pain	Any pain that has occurred within the past 7 days
Recent problem	A problem arising in the last week

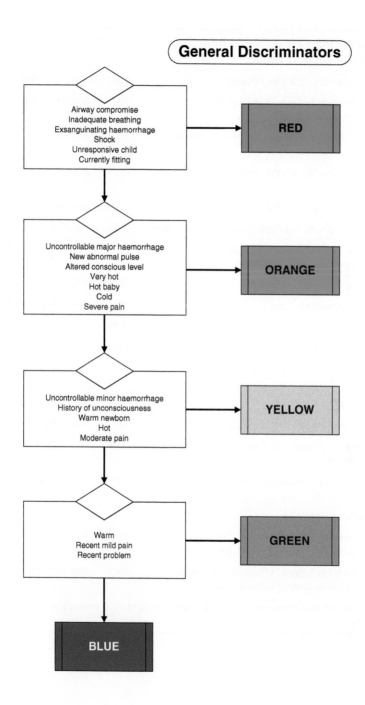

General Discriminators

The following titles are available from the Advanced Life Support Group:

Paediatric and Neonatal Critical Care Transport	2003	9780727917706
Major Incident Medical Management and Support: The Practical Approach in the Hospital	2005	9780727918680
Safe Transfer and Retrieval of Patients: The Practical Approach, 2nd Edition	2006	9780727918550
Paediatric and Neonatal Safe Transfer and Retrieval: The Practical Approach	2008	9781405169196
Pre-hospital Obstetric Emergency Training	2009	9781405184755
Acute Medical Emergencies: The Practical Approach, 2nd Edition	2010	9780727918543
Major Incident Medical Management and Support: The Practical Approach at the Scene, 3rd Edition	2011	9781405187572
Human Factors in the Healthcare Setting	2013	9781118339701
Comprehensive Tracheostomy Care	2014	9781118792773
Emergency Triage, 3rd Edition	2014	9781118299067
Telephone Triage and Advice	2014	9781118369388
Hazardous Incident Medical Management and Support: The Practical Approach	2015	9780727914637
Paediatric Emergency Triage	2015	9781118299012
Pocket Guide to Teaching for Clinical Instructors, 3rd Edition	2015	9781118860076
Advanced Paediatric Life Support: A Practical Approach to Emergencies, 6th Edition	2016	9781118947647
Pre-Hospital Paediatric Life Support: A Practical Approach to Emergencies, 3rd Edition	2017	9781118339763

Australia and NZ Adaptations

Australasian Disaster Management: incorporating Major Incident Medical Management and Support, 3rd edition	2013	9780470657751
Advanced Paediatric Life Support: A Practical Approach to Emergencies, 6th Edition Australia and New Zealand	2017	9781119385462

Each of these titles has an accompanying course – to learn more about ALSG courses visit **www.alsg.org**